Risk Management

Clinical, Ethical, & Legal Guidelines for Successful Practice

William F. Doverspike

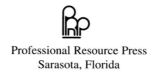

Professional Resource Press
Sarasota, Florida

Published by
Professional Resource Press
(An Imprint of the Professional Resource Exchange, Inc.)
Post Office Box 3197
Sarasota, FL 34230-3197

Printed in the United States of America

The copy editor for this book was Patricia Rockwood, the managing editor was Debbie Fink, the production coordinator was Laurie Girsch, and the cover designer was Stacey Sanders.

Library of Congress Cataloging-in-Publication Data

Doverspike, William F., 1951-
   Risk management : clinical, ethical, & legal guidelines for successful practice / William F. Doverspike.
    p. ; cm.
   Includes bibliographical references and indexes.
   ISBN-13: 978-1-56887-108-0 (alk. paper)
   ISBN-10: 1-56887-108-2 (alk. paper)
  1. Medical ethics. 2. Risk management. I. Title.
   [DNLM: 1. Ethics, Clinical. 2. Ethics, Medical. 3. Risk Management. WB 60 D743r 2008]
   R725.5.D68 2008
   174.2--dc22

                            2007038419

Acknowledgments

Writing an ethics book is more than researching ethical standards and case law. It is about sharing the knowledge and skills that have been shared with me by those who have shaped my career. There are several people who, by teaching me how to put ethics into practice, laid the foundation for *Risk Management: Clinical, Ethical, and Legal Guidelines for Successful Practice.*

I thank my colleagues in the Georgia Psychological Association (GPA), particularly those who have served with me on the Ethics Committee, for their wisdom, support, and encouragement over the years. For over a decade, many colleagues have consulted with me about ethical dilemmas that have required us to collaborate and discover solutions to problems that no one of us could have discovered alone.

I thank my colleagues Ted Ballard, PhD, Tom Friedrichs, PhD, and Linda Scott, PhD, for being role models who encouraged me to strive for excellence early in my career. These are the colleagues who I often envisioned when faced with difficult ethical dilemmas early in my career. Later in my career, when I was elected President of GPA, Ted became a trusted advisor who reminded me of the importance of thinking collaboratively, striving for humility, and listening to others before making important decisions.

I thank Rob Remar, Esquire, for providing valuable legal consultations that provided a foundation for my interests in ethical risk management. Rob stood beside me during one of the most difficult trials I have ever faced. I thank my brother David Doverspike, Esquire, for teaching me to think like a lawyer in terms of liability risk management, and to think like a doctor in terms of clinical management and patient care. As a brother, David has been a role model who lives by moral principles, and as a lawyer David has often reminded me that I protect myself by protecting my patients first. I thank my friend the late Honorable Robin Nash for helping me learn to do the next right thing when making ethical decisions.

Robin taught me that sometimes the best response option was doing nothing at all. I thank my friend and advisor, Craig Mullins, for encouraging me to put my ideas into writing in the form of a book. I began writing the original edition of *Ethical Risk Management: Guidelines for Practice* shortly after one of our meetings 10 years ago.

I thank Eric Harris, EdD, JD, for inspiring me with his sharp intellect and quick wit that have always made his ethics seminars entertaining as well as enlightening. I thank Jeff Younggren, PhD, for his commonsense reasoning and sense of humor, as well as for his personal encouragement over the years. Jeff's video clips have added a stimulating dimension to my lectures in ethics classes. The reader will notice that throughout this book I frequently quote the advice that Drs. Younggren and Harris provide in their liability risk management seminars sponsored by the American Psychological Association Insurance Trust (APAIT).

I thank the late George Taylor, PhD, for giving me the opportunity to teach my first ethics class, an experience that changed the direction of my career. I thank the great Linda Campbell, PhD, for referring to me as an ethics professor before I even became one. As one of my mentors, Linda saw in me what I could not see in myself and, in doing so, she helped me become a better teacher to my own students. I thank my colleague Jeff Terrell, PhD, for providing me the opportunity to teach professional ethics in a faith-based counseling program, where I had the honor of witnessing virtue ethics and principle ethics being integrated as a way of life. I thank my students at the Psychological Studies Institute (PSI) in Atlanta for constantly challenging me to practice what I preach. I thank my students at Argosy University for asking questions that have inspired me to increase my knowledge of ethics.

I thank several of my friends for their support of my work in the field of ethics. I thank my colleague Susan Reid, LCSW, for being available for our hallway consultations that have occurred on a regular basis over the years. Susan has often helped me see my ethical blind spots at times when other colleagues have simply told me to keep up the good work. I thank my friend and colleague Joanne Peeler, RN, PhD, for the support she has always given to me when I have been nervous or uncertain of myself when presenting professional seminars to colleagues. Joanne often reminded me that a good ethics teacher lies somewhere on the continuum between Moses and Cool Hand Luke. I thank my friend Deborah Midkiff, MS, for the positive influence she has had on me through the intentionality by which she lives her faith. Deborah has been inspirational to me as a faith-based counselor whose professional practice and personal life are based on integrating moral principles as a way of life.

I thank several of my brothers, whose anonymity I will protect by not mentioning them by name, in the Saturday Morning Men's Meeting for their ongoing communal support of my personal efforts to live by principles rather than by personalities. I thank my fellow professors in the Saturday afternoon Sabbath Smokers, including Ricks Carson, Steve Fowler, John Offerdahl, and Tedd Weitzman, for their enlightening exchange of ideas that have sharpened my skills as a teacher and, more importantly, as a student of ethics.

I thank Cyd Wise, managing editor of the *Georgia Psychologist* magazine, for the experience, strength, and hope that she has shared with me over the years. The original edition of *Ethical Risk Management* was essentially a collection of some of the ethics articles I had published in the *Georgia Psychologist*.

I thank Laura Hahn for her assistance in reading the final galley proofs. She demonstrated a standard of excellence through her meticulous attention to detail.

Last but not least, I thank my colleagues at Professional Resource Press for actually publishing my book. Larry and Jude Ritt have been supportive of my work ever since they first published my early ethics articles in their encyclopedia of practice resources known as *Innovations in Clinical Practice*. In particular, I thank Debbie Fink, managing editor for Professional Resource Press, for helping me improve my writing skills over the years. Each time I grade the papers of my students or edit the articles of my peers, I appreciate the skills that Debbie taught me. I would also like to thank Laurie Girsch, production coordinator, for her assistance. Together, they turned my manuscript into a book.

I dedicate this book to my father and my mother, who gave me my first ethics book.

Preface

When I was invited to become a member of my state professional association's Ethics Committee, I agreed to do so after learning that the committee's role had become more educative and less adjudicative in its functions. At my first committee meeting, I quickly discovered that the vast majority of my colleagues were careful, conscientious, and compassionate in their work. If you are reading this book, you are probably a member of that vast majority. If you regularly consult with colleagues about what you are doing, you are definitely one of those careful and conscientious practitioners.

While investigating complaints for the state Ethics Committee, I was also surprised and somewhat perplexed to learn that the most serious ethical violations could have been avoided in the first place had the practitioner simply observed some of the most basic ethical principles. I noticed that the most serious violations could have been prevented altogether had the practitioner simply followed the most fundamental guidelines such as "always practice within your area of competence" and "maintain clear boundaries." In cases in which clients alleged less serious complaints, the practice of "keeping current with standards" and "consulting with a colleague" were particularly relevant. In situations involving unfounded complaints, a well-documented record was always the best defense.

As I began to review more and more cases, I was impressed with how often the same ethical principles applied to different situations. I began to compile a list of some practical guidelines based on these observations. Most of these guidelines are not ethical principles but rather are simply some commonsense strategies for putting ethics into practice. These practical guidelines focus more on what to do rather than on what not to do. It's what I call Ethics 101.

In providing consultations to colleagues who have faced complex situations in which no single course of ethical action seemed clear, I began to understand the importance of using a problem-solving or decision-making model in applying ethical standards to specific situations. Finally, when reviewing office procedures of colleagues who seemed to aspire to ethical excellence, I developed a greater appreciation for the use of informed consent procedures and good documentation practices that help prevent ethical problems before they arise. In my opinion, most ethical problems can be prevented when practitioners use good communication, consultation, and documentation.

These basic guidelines provide the framework for *Ethical Risk Management: Guidelines for Practice*, the revision of which has been expanded as *Risk Management: Clinical, Ethical, and Legal Guidelines for Successful Practice*. Incorporating these practical guidelines and decision-making models into your practice patterns may offer you a greater degree of protection while you offer your clients a higher standard of care. Remember, when you protect your patient, you protect yourself.

William F. Doverspike, PhD, ABPP
Atlanta, Georgia
January 2008

Table of Contents

ACKNOWLEDGMENTS   iii

PREFACE   vii

CONTENTS OF THE CD-ROM   xiii

HOW TO USE THE CD-ROM   xxiii

CHAPTER ONE
Ethical Risk Management:
Some Personal Reflections   1

Understand Ethical and Legal Standards   3
Practice Within Your Area of Competence   4
Supervise Only What You Know   8
Obtain Adequate Informed Consent   9
Be Aware of Child Custody Evaluations   11
Maintain Clear Boundaries With Clients   13
Use Projective Retrospective Thinking   14
Consult With a Colleague   15
Document Your Decisions in Writing   16
Keep Communication Channels Open   18
Aspire to a Standard of Excellence   20
An Alternative View: The Myth of Risk Management   21
Summary of Ethical Risk-Management Considerations   23
Points to Remember   24

CHAPTER TWO
Informed Consent Considerations:
Preventing Ethical Problems Before They Arise   25

An Overview of Informed Consent   26
Understand the Ethical Principles   27
Determine Capacity to Consent   28
Provide Significant Information   29
Avoid Undue Influence   33
Obtain Written Documentation   34
Note Exceptions to Informed Consent   35
Consider Legal Standards   38
Consider Federal Regulations   39
Consider Managed Care   40
Use Informed Consent Forms   41
Summary of Informed Consent Considerations   43
Points to Remember   44

CHAPTER THREE
Managing Boundaries:
Staying Off the Slippery Slope   45

Dual Relationships   46
Risk Factors and Unhealthy Boundaries   59
Sexual Impropriety   61
Special Considerations   65
Summary of Managing Boundaries   80
Points to Remember   81

CHAPTER FOUR
Ethical Decision Making:
Doing the Next Right Thing   83

Principle Ethics and Virtue Ethics   85
Teleological and Deontological Ethics   86
Some Basic Decision-Making Models   88
An Ethical Decision-Making Model   94
Identifying Conflicts Between Ethical and Legal Guidelines 108
Psychology and the Law   109
Solving Ethical Problems Before They Arise   110
Summary of Decision-Making Guidelines   111
Points to Remember   112

CHAPTER FIVE
Consulting With Colleagues:
Don't Worry Alone 113

Common Ethical Dichotomies 115
Top 10 Reasons Not to Consult a Colleague 118
Top 10 Reasons to Consult a Colleague 120
Psychological Versus Legal Consultations 168
Summary of Consulting With Colleagues 170
Points to Remember 171

CHAPTER SIX
Documentation and Record Keeping:
Putting It in Writing 173

Record Retention 174
Child Records 177
Psychotherapy Notes 180
Progress Notes 181
Risk-Managed Notes 184
Summary of Records 185
Disclosure of Information 187
Client Access 188
Written Reports 189
Summary of Documentation and Record Keeping 191
Points to Remember 191

CHAPTER SEVEN
Responding Ethically to Complaints and
Investigations: Turning Negatives into Positives 193

Responding to the Notice of Investigation 194
There is No Such Thing as a Frivolous Complaint 194
Be a Colleague, Not an Adversary 195
Be a Behaviorist When Explaining Details 195
Explain in Writing What You Did and Why You Did It 196
Be Sure to Cite the Standards 196
Do Not Blame the Client 197
Put Principles Before Personalities 197
Learn How to Turn Errors into Amends 198
Show Concern for Your Client's Welfare 198
Note Any Peer Consultations 198

CHAPTER SEVEN
Responding Ethically to Complaints and
Investigations: Turning Negatives into Positives *(Cont'd)*

Think In Terms of Aspirational Behavior   199
Be Aware of Procedures and Deadlines   199
Understand the Committee Findings   200
Turn a Negative into a Positive   201
Summary of Responding to Ethics Complaints   201
Points to Remember   202

REFERENCES   203

SUBJECT INDEX   221

AUTHOR INDEX   233

LIST OF TABLES

Table 1: Types of Dual Relationships   50
Table 2: Examples of Types of Therapist Disclosures   66
Table 3: Types of Special Events   77
Table 4: The 2 x 2 Factorial Matrix   91
Table 5: Differences Between Test Data and Test Materials   138

Contents of
the CD-ROM

The CD-ROM includes a series of sample consent forms on a variety of topics ranging from A to Z and beyond. These consent forms and practice policies are not intended to provide legal advice, and the information contained in them should not be relied upon for legal advice. The reader is encouraged to contact a qualified attorney for legal advice regarding state and federal laws governing informed consent.

Form 1: An *Office Policies and Procedures* form. Although not serving as a protocol for office policies, the brief form provides some useful information to new and prospective clients. The information contained in this form can be placed on the practitioner's website or mailed to callers or prospective clients who are contemplating counseling services. This form is listed first in order to emphasize the central theme of creating reasonable client expectations in advance.

Form 2: A *Client Registration* form. This form is listed early in the series because most mental health professionals begin the intake process by having the client complete a client registration form, also known as a client information sheet. However, it is a good ethical practice to discuss informed consent considerations, including the exceptions to confidentiality, before the client discloses any personal information. Such a practice protects the client's right to privacy before he or she provides any personal information.

Form 3: An *Informed Consent Checklist*. This form was designed for clinicians choosing an informal approach to informed consent considerations. The checklist serves as a reminder for the mental health professional to discuss office policies; benefits, risks, and alternatives to treatment; exceptions of privacy, privilege, and confidentiality; and other information that may be appropriate over the course of therapy. The checklist includes some items, such as the use of innovative, risky, or unusual techniques, which may be applicable to some practitioners and not to others.

Form 4: An *Informed Consent for Psychological Services* form. This form is designed for clinicians who prefer a more formal approach than the use of an informal checklist. The consent form contains information that addresses clinical services related to scope of practice, assumption of risks and benefits, limits of confidentiality, and the release of information. Because the original version of this form was designed for my hospital practice that includes diagnostic consultations, there is an emphasis on the release of information to the referral source. For this reason, the reader is encouraged to modify the content so that it is more suitable for other purposes. Although it is easy for practitioners to lapse into unethical habits such as having clients "sign-off" on consent forms, the use of client initials on various sections of the consent form often facilitates discussion with the client during the process of informed consent.

Form 5: An *Informed Consent for Financial Responsibility* form. Although many clinicians use one large consent form that combines clinical and financial information, there are times when separate forms may be useful (e.g., when the client and the guarantor of payment are not the same person). The financial consent form contains information related to financial responsibility, fees for services, insurance filing, financial arrangements, managed care contracts, guarantee of payment, billing and collections, and release of information for third-party payments. Again, the use of client initials on various sections of the consent form often facilitates discussion and encourages the client to ask questions regarding any information that he or she does not fully understand.

Form 6: A *Statement of Understanding for Unauthorized Services and for Services Beyond Medical Necessity* form. This form is actually another type of financial consent form, which emphasizes that there are some services that are not covered or reimbursed under health insurance plans or managed care plans. The form is particularly important for managed care clients requesting services that are either unauthorized by the managed care company, beyond the scope of coverage of the policy, or may not meet medical necessity criteria. The form can also be used with managed care clients who prefer to self-pay for their care in order to protect their privacy interests. The form is simply a way to provide documentation of a client's understanding and agreement under these limited circumstances.

Form 7: A *Statement of Understanding for Appointments That Are Unkept, Canceled, or Rescheduled With Less Than 24 Hours' Notice* form. Although most mental health professionals clearly state their "no-show" policy within the language of their general consent form, the late cancelation policy is one of the most frequently forgotten policies by clients the first time a late cancelation or "rescheduling" request occurs. For this reason, it is often helpful to ensure that the client clearly understands the practitioner's cancelation policy in advance.

Form 8: A *Statement of Understanding for Telephone Conferences* form. Although clients routinely call offices of professionals for various reasons, this consent form can serve as an additional reminder to specific clients who use the phone for extended crisis-intervention calls. Some clients reduce their scheduled therapy visits and then use the phone for between-session consultations with the therapist. Although telephone support is an intervention that is used in some empirically supported treatment paradigms (e.g., dialectical behavior therapy), the use of a formal written agreement can help to reduce any misunderstandings if the therapist has a policy of charging for phone conferences. The form is not designed as a substitute for sound clinical management of boundaries, but rather is used as a way of documenting an agreement between therapist and client.

Form 9: A *Record of Phone Conversation* form. Particularly for therapists using the phone as an adjunct to treatment sessions, a phone log or record of conversation is as important as a progress note. Of course, there is no reason to document a phone consultation using a separate type of note, but the Record of Phone Conversation is designed simply as a reminder for the conscientious therapist to document all phone contacts with clients.

Form 10: A *Consultation Note* form. Such a note can be used for a variety of purposes, ranging from documentation of an initial assessment interview to a consultation with a colleague. Because the initial assessment interview or intake interview does not necessarily involve treatment, but in fact may result in a referral or other disposition of the client, there may be some precedent for documenting the intake interview differently than a therapy session. For example, an intake interview may lead to career counseling or psychological testing, which would be documented in subsequent consultation notes or a psychological report. Alternatively, an intake interview may lead to psychotherapy, which would later be documented in a Progress Note or Psychotherapy Note. In addition, a Consultation Note can be used to document consultations with other mental health professionals. Practitioners are generally in the habit of documenting their intake evaluations, but they often do not document their consultations with colleagues. For this reason, the Consultation Note serves as a reminder of the importance of not only consulting with peers but also documenting such consultations.

Form 11: A *Progress Note* form. In general, practitioners should write behaviorally oriented progress notes rather than interpretively oriented process notes. The note is obviously not any different than the Consultation Note, but the difference lies in the fact that the Consultation Note does not imply that treatment is necessarily being contemplated or occurring, whereas the Progress Note represents an explicit documentation of the progress of treatment.

Form 12: A *Psychotherapy Note* form. Although this note is essentially the same as the preceding notes except for the heading, the differences among the headings are significant. In light of state and federal laws governing privileged communication, one may need reminding that it is specifically *psychotherapeutic* communication (e.g., *Jaffee v. Redmond*, 1996) that is protected from forced disclosure in court and in legal proceedings. For this reason, the conscientious practitioner affords his or her client a greater degree of privacy protection by clearly specifying what is and what is not psychotherapeutic communication. In addition, federal HIPAA regulations also afford a higher degree of privacy protection for notes that are segregated from the clinical record and that meet the specific

HIPAA definition of "Psychotherapy Notes." However, most ethicists and legal analysts recommend keeping progress notes and maintaining one set of records rather than two sets.

Form 13: A *Client History* form. Although this type of form would not be appropriate for all practitioners, I used the form for many years when providing hospital consultations because it allowed a way to write brief narrative notes when reviewing hospital charts and when interviewing patients. I would typically jot down some notes on the form while reviewing the hospitalized patient's chart, and then later add some more notes when interviewing the patient. When obtaining information from different sources (e.g., patient-report, chart review, or collateral interview data), the source of information should be specified on the form. Although the order of items in the form might seem somewhat arbitrary, the format provided an organizational template for the first half of my psychological reports. I would simply dictate information into the psychological report that followed the basic order of the form, which provided a relatively efficient and standardized way of writing reports.

Form 14: A *Client Background Information* form. This form can be completed by the client prior to the intake appointment or during the appointment itself. It can also be used by the practitioner when taking notes during the intake session. The best practice would probably include having the client complete the form prior to the intake appointment and then having the practitioner add some clarification notes during the intake interview. If information is obtained from or supplemented by other sources (e.g., medical records, collateral informant), then the name of the informant or the source of the information should be specified on the form. While the choice and order of items on the form might seem somewhat arbitrary, the format provides some basic information that may be useful during the assessment stage of individual psychotherapy.

Form 15: A *Mental Status Examination* form. The narrative approach is not as quick and efficient as the checklist approach, which uses forms that contain boxes and squares that simply need to be checked. However, the narrative approach is more flexible in that it encourages a more verbal description of mental status in the therapist's own words.

Form 16: A *Problem List* form. The form can be used as part of a homework assignment to help a client conceptualize and operationalize a short problem list. The simple rating scale allows the client and therapist to measure changes and outcome at a later point in time.

Form 17: A *Treatment Plan Worksheet* form. This form can be used to transform problems into goals and then translate goals into the specific objectives needed to attain them.

Form 18: A *Behavioral Changes Worksheet* form. This form represents an approach that is not any different from the Treatment Plan Worksheet, which essentially evolved into the Behavioral Changes Worksheet when I first began working with clients in a way that focused more on normality and less on pathology.

Form 19: A *Commitment to Treatment* form. This form has been used, adapted, and modified by permission of the American Psychological Association Insurance Trust (APAIT). Permission was also obtained from David Rudd, the original author of the form used in the APAIT workshops. Modifications to the form were based on the APAIT's Model Crisis Response Plan form presented in Younggren's (2006, pp. 26-27) handouts.

Form 20: A *Collaterals Consent Form.* This form has been used, adapted, and modified by permission of the American Psychological Association Insurance Trust (APAIT). The form provides information that clarifies the role of the collateral, and the form helps manage expectations by explaining that the collateral is not the client. The original form may be downloaded from the APAIT website.

Form 21: A *Policy on Sharing Information About Child Clients With Courts* form. The form has been used, adapted, and modified by permission of the American Psychological Association Insurance Trust (APAIT).

Form 22: An *Informed Consent for Special Circumstances: Couples and Family Therapy* form. The purpose of this form is to clarify the policy of sharing information received individually from either participant with the other participant so that the therapist is not placed in a position of triangulation. The form also informs the participants that any releases of confidential information require the written consent of both parties.

Form 23: An *Informed Consent for Special Circumstances: Children and Adolescents Ages 15 and Under* form. The purpose of this form is to clarify that consent for treatment of a minor child must be obtained from both parents unless there is some legal custody agreement that has been documented. The form also acknowledges that parents have the right of access to information about their child, and that the therapist will use professional judgment regarding balancing the parents' legal right to information and the child's ethical right to privacy of specific communications in therapy.

Form 24: An *Informed Consent for Special Circumstances: Adolescents Ages 16 to 17 Years Old* form. The purpose of this form is to manage expectations at the outset by clarifying the therapist's confidentiality policy with respect to therapy with mature minors. The form also states one of the ethically justifiable exceptions to confidentiality in the case of dangerousness to self or others.

Form 25: An *Informed Consent for Special Circumstances: Young Adults Ages 18 Years and Older* form. The form states a confidentiality policy that would be typical when working with competent adult clients who are entitled to the rights of confidentiality. The form states an ethically justifiable exception to confidentiality in the case of dangerousness to self or others.

Form 26: An *Informed Consent for Psychological Testing* form. The form explains psychological testing in a brief way that demystifies testing and helps reduce a client's anxiety prior to undergoing a psychological evaluation. This form is given to clients who are contemplating testing; the form is often mailed to prospective clients who have called with questions about testing.

Form 27: An *Informed Consent for Neuropsychological Testing* form. Essentially the same as the Informed Consent for Psychological Testing form from which it was derived, the Informed Consent for Neuropsychological Testing form simply explains the process of cognitive and neuropsychological testing in plain English. This form is also mailed to prospective clients before they undergo testing.

Form 28: An *Informed Consent for Counseling and Psychotherapy* form. The form simply helps create reasonable expectations on the part of the client. The form emphasizes an active collaborative approach to counseling and psychotherapy, briefly mentions some possible benefits and risks of psychotherapy, and provides information for consideration of treatment alternatives to psychotherapy.

Form 29: An *Informed Consent for Termination of Professional Services* form. This form is not used with all clients, but it may be useful with clients for whom termination should be carefully discussed in advance. The form provides a brief description of some of the ethical justifications for termination as well as the ethical means by which the process of termination will be conducted.

Form 30: An *Informed Consent for Independent Consultative Examination* form. The purpose of this form is to clearly identify the organizational client, clarify the practitioner's role, and create realistic expectations on the part of the person being evaluated. The form clearly states to the person being evaluated that he or she may not be entitled to receive an explanation of the assessment results.

Form 31: A *Sample Letter of Agreement Regarding Financial Responsibility for Expert Testimony*. The form letter provides a template for documenting a financial agreement with an attorney who wishes to retain a practitioner for expert testimony. The form clarifies the practitioner's scope of services and thereby creates realistic expectations on the part of the attorney.

Form 32: A *Sample Letter for Response to Request for Production of Documents*. The purpose of the form letter is to acknowledge receipt of a Request for Production of Documents and to assert privilege. The user is encouraged to consult with an attorney and to cite the appropriate legal statutes of the state in which the licensed mental health professional is licensed to practice.

Form 33: A *Sample Letter for Response to Subpoena (for Licensed Psychologists)*. The letter asserts privilege in response to a subpoena for psychotherapy records for which the client has not authorized disclosure. The form letter clarifies that psychotherapy communications are privileged as defined by state and federal laws. The user is encouraged to consult with an attorney and to cite the appropriate legal statutes of the state in which the licensed mental health professional is licensed to practice.

Form 34: A *Sample Letter for Response to Subpoena (for Licensed Professional Counselors)*. The letter asserts privilege in response to a subpoena for psychotherapy records for which the client has not authorized disclosure. The form letter clarifies that psychotherapy communications are privileged as defined by state and federal laws. The user is encouraged to consult with an attorney and to cite the appropriate legal statutes of the state in which the licensed mental health professional is licensed to practice.

Form 35: A *Waiver of Privilege* form for documenting the client's waiver of the psychotherapist-patient privilege and authorization for the release of psychological report. The form can be used with clients who request testimony in court.

Form 36: A *Telephone Reply to Telephone Request for Information* about a client or former client. The form is simply a reminder of how patient privacy can be protected when returning phone calls. Of course, if a therapist receives a phone call from a person requesting confidential information in the absence of a signed, written authorization, one option is to consider not returning the call in the first place.

Form 37: A *Release of Information Form* for the release of confidential information. The authorization form specifies the name of the person to whom the information will be released, the specific nature of the information, and the specific purpose of the disclosure.

Form 38: A HIPAA-compliant *Authorization Form* for the release of protected health information (PHI). The authorization form specifies the information to be disclosed, the name of the person to whom the information is to be disclosed, the specific purpose of the disclosure (if applicable), the effective date and expiration date of the disclosure, and the right to revoke the authorization.

Form 39: A *Closing Summary*. The note is similar in function to a counseling Termination Note or a hospital Discharge Summary Note, all of which indicate the date of termination and the circumstances around which professional services have been completed. The note serves as a reminder of the importance of documenting termination of treatment from a liability risk-management perspective. In other words: no patient; no liability.

Form 40: A *Treatment Outcome Measure*. The survey can be used as a simple measure of the client's posttreatment level of functioning and as a formal way of following up with former clients.

Form 41: A *Client Satisfaction Survey*. The survey can be used as a simple measure of the client's satisfaction with the services received.

Form 42: A *Professional Plan for the Sudden Termination of Practice.* After all is said and done, the only thing that remains to be done is making preparation for the handling of one's practice in the event of a termination of one's professional practice. This form has been used, adapted, and modified by permission of the North Carolina Society for Clinical Social Work (NCSCSW). The Professional Plan for the Sudden Termination of Practice form was developed from NCSCSW's pamphlet/ brochure, "A Suggested Model for the Sudden Termination of a Clinical Social Work Practice." The original form may be obtained directly from NCSCSW. The form addresses such topics as client notification, physician notification, retention and disposition of client records, and other information. Pope and Vasquez (2005) also provide information concerning a "Therapist's Guide for Preparing a Professional Will." Chapter 8 of Pope and Vasquez contains a 17-step guide that can be used in creating a professional will.

The CD-ROM also includes a PowerPoint® file containing slides that provide an outline of the chapters of *Risk Management: Clinical, Ethical, and Legal Guidelines for Successful Practice.* Each chapter is outlined by key concepts, major sections, minor headings, and points to remember. The file can be used to print handouts and create presentations for use in the classroom and in ethics seminars. The file may be easily modified by the user to suit his or her instructional needs.

How to Use the CD-ROM

INTRODUCTION

The material on this CD-ROM is saved as Adobe Portable Document Format (PDF) files. In order to use this material, you will need to have software capable of reading Adobe Portable Document Format (PDF) files.

SYSTEM REQUIREMENTS

If you have *Adobe Reader* installed on your computer, this CD-ROM may be used with most versions of the Windows operating system as well as most versions of MacOS, Linux, Palm OS, and Pocket PC. A free version of *Adobe Reader* may be downloaded at the *Adobe Reader* website:

http://www.adobe.com/products/acrobat/readstep2.html

That site also contains detailed information about system requirements for using the software, a downloadable user's guide, user's forums, and other useful information. Most users find that simply downloading the software enables them to open and use PDF files such as those included on the CD-ROM.

HOW TO INSTALL AND USE THE FILES

After *Adobe Reader* is installed, you can copy the contents of the CD-ROM to a convenient place on your hard disk and each file should open automatically when you click on it. You can identify Adobe Portable Document Format files because they all have a PDF extension (e.g.,

Sample.pdf). If Windows asks you to choose a program to open the file with, choose Adobe Reader 8.1 (or the latest version).

Adobe Reader allows you to print exact reproductions of the material on the CD-ROM to the printer(s) installed on your computer; however, it will not allow you to edit or modify the materials. If you want to edit or modify the material, you will need to order one of Adobe's other products from www.adobe.com or http://www.adobe.com/products/acrobat/readstep2.html (e.g., Adobe Acrobat 8 Professional).

PERMISSION TO USE THIS MATERIAL

Purchasers of this product have the unlimited right to print copies of the materials on this CD-ROM for use with their clients. However, they may not share copies of either this CD-ROM or the materials contained herein with others without explicit written consent from the publisher, Professional Resource Exchange, Inc.

Risk Management

Clinical, Ethical, & Legal Guidelines for Successful Practice

Chapter One

Ethical Risk Management: Some Personal Reflections

Dear Reader:

The State Licensing Board would like to meet with you at an informal fact-finding inquiry before members of the Board's Investigative Committee.

Please be advised that your participation in this proceeding is strictly voluntary, and that your failure to appear will not be used against you at a formal hearing and will not be an admission to any wrongdoing. If you choose to appear, any statements you make or information gathered may be used against you at a formal hearing and may be further used by the Board in determining what sanctions, if any, may be appropriate in your case. You may appear with or without an attorney. After an investigative interview is held, the Board may determine that an informal disposition of the case is appropriate or may decide that no action is warranted. If you decline to accept the Board's informal disposition, a formal hearing may be scheduled.

The Board would like to schedule an investigative interview at the Board office. Upon receipt of this letter, please immediately telephone and advise me as to whether you will attend, and I will then schedule a date and time for you.

Sincerely yours,

Board Secretary

A variation on the theme of the form letter on the preceding page might be your first notice that a licensing board complaint has been filed against you. Because the prime directive of state licensing boards is to protect the public, you may be required to cooperate in an investigation without being informed of the name of the person who filed the complaint. In some cases, you may be required to defend a complaint without even knowing the nature of the complaint. At its sole discretion, the licensing board may expand the investigation to include other areas of your practice, an investigative process that is sometimes referred to as a "fishing expedition." After you have spent considerable time, money, and energy addressing the complaint, the licensing board will render a verdict that may have implications regarding your future employability, insurability, and marketability.

Now that I have your attention, I would like to introduce you to a practical handbook that addresses ethics from a risk-management perspective. For those who do not wish to take the time to read the book, the basic idea is that ethical problems can be prevented through the use of common sense. One of the problems, however, is that practitioners sometimes do not use commonsense principles. These principles include practicing within your area of competence, using an ongoing process of informed consent to create realistic client expectations in advance, managing boundaries appropriately, consulting with colleagues when in doubt about a course of action, and maintaining good record keeping and documentation.

For those who do wish to read the book, I will use personal observations written from a first-person perspective to provide you with an informal discussion of some practical guidelines designed to help colleagues integrate ethical principles into their clinical work.* In other words, it is a book about putting ethics into practice. Because I practice as a psychologist, most of the material is written from a psychological perspective, although the ethical guidelines are general enough that they are not confined to any specific profession. Because this book is written for mental health professionals (MHP), the terms psychotherapist, counselor, clinician, and provider are often used interchangeably. Similarly, although there are some specific differences between the terms

---

* Although the principles contained in this book are applicable to all mental health pro- fessionals, the author acknowledges that psychologists, psychiatrists, social workers, marriage and family therapists, and professional counselors have different ethics codes, licensing board rules, and specialty guidelines that they follow. This book is not intended to provide legal advice, and the information contained in it should not be relied upon for legal advice. The reader is encouraged to contact a qualified attorney for legal advice regarding state laws governing professional conduct.

client and *patient* (e.g., the term patient has a medical connotation and is often used to refer to someone undergoing psychotherapy, whereas the term client is more general and is often used to refer to someone receiving counseling), the two terms are often used interchangeably. The text of this handbook is based on three chapters that originally appeared in *Innovations in Clinical Practice* (Doverspike, 1995, 1997b, 1999c) as well as a series of ethics articles that originally appeared in the *Georgia Psychologist* magazine (Doverspike, 1996a, 1996b, 1997a, 1997c, 1999a, 1999e, 2000, 2001, 2003a, 2003b, 2004b, 2005c, 2005d, 2006b, 2006c, 2006d).

UNDERSTAND ETHICAL
AND LEGAL STANDARDS

Sometimes we err without realizing what we are doing, only later to learn that ignorance of the law is a poor defense. Perhaps the place to start is with your profession's Code of Ethics itself, because such codes are often incorporated into the statutory laws of many states.* A good rule of thumb is to be sure you have a copy of your profession's Code of Ethics and your state licensing board's Code of Conduct so that these can be consulted from time to time. When confronting an ethical dilemma, just refreshing your memory by reviewing relevant standards can help improve your ethical decision-making process. If a single relevant standard applies in a particular situation, then your first question should be, "Is there a reason to deviate from the standard?" (Haas & Malouf, 2005, p. 12).

For psychologists, the applicable Ethics Code is the American Psychological Association (APA; 2002) *Ethical Principles of Psychologists and Code of Conduct*, often referred to as simply the Ethics Code. For psychiatrists, the applicable code is the American Psychiatric Association (2001) *The Principles of Medical Ethics With Annotations Especially Applicable to Psychiatry*. For social workers, there is the National Association of Social Workers (NASW; 1999) *Code of Ethics*. For marriage and family therapists, the relevant code is the American Association for Marriage and Family Therapy (AAMFT; 2001) *Code of Ethics*. For counselors, the applicable code is the American Counseling Association (ACA; 2005) *Code of Ethics*, hereafter referred to as simply the Code of Ethics. For those interested in maintaining the highest standard

---

* The APA Ethics Code is codified into the licensing board rules and regulations of approximately 27 states.

of care, consider reading one of the commentaries on the various Codes of Ethics. For psychologists, ethics commentaries and case studies include *Ethics for Psychologists: A Commentary on the APA Ethics Code* (Canter et al., 1994) and *Ethical Conflicts in Psychology* (Bersoff, 2003). For professional counselors, particularly those who are members of the ACA, ethics commentaries and case studies are provided in the *American Counseling Association Ethical Standards Casebook* (Herlihy & G. Corey, 2006).

Consider having a discussion with a respected colleague regarding a section of the Ethics Code that is relevant to your common areas of practice. Have a *scenario-based* discussion rather than a *procedure-based* conference. In other words, rather than taking an ethical standard and discussing all the situations in which it may apply, try taking a potentially problematic clinical situation and discussing all of the ethical standards that may apply. Ask questions. What are the differences between privacy, privilege, and confidentiality? Under what circumstances is privilege abrogated? How do you obtain informed consent from a client whose competence is in question? Does a client's authorization for release of confidential information always have to be in writing? How much information does a managed care patient require in order to give informed consent? Who owns and controls the privilege of a deceased patient's psychotherapy records?

Clinicians interested in improving their ethical decision-making abilities may also be interested in reviewing the literature on decision-making models (e.g., G. Corey, M. Corey, & Callanan, 2007; Eberlein, 1987; Haas & Malouf, 2005; Hill, Glaser, & Harden, 1995; Keith-Spiegel & Koocher, 1985; Kitchener, 1984; Koocher & Keith-Spiegel, 1998; Remley & Herlihy, 2005; Welfel, 2006). These models typically include several steps that typify ethical decision making, including identification of relevant issues and practices, identification of applicable ethical standards, development of alternative courses of action, analysis of likely risks and benefits of each course of action, and evaluation of the results of the course of action. Some of these models are discussed in greater detail later in this book in the chapter on Ethical Decision Making (Chapter 4, pp. 83-112).

PRACTICE WITHIN YOUR
AREA OF COMPETENCE

Many times when a licensing board investigates ethics complaints, the first area of inquiry involves the standard of *competence*. For example, in the investigation of a complaint in which one partner in couples counseling has accused the counselor of breaking the confidentiality of that partner's disclosure made privately during a phone call to the counselor, one initial area of inquiry (also known as an "informal fact-finding inquiry") may involve whether the couples counselor is qualified or competent to provide couples counseling in the first place. In other words, the investigation may be expanded beyond the initial complaint by examining the ethical issue of competence as well as the actual complaint alleged by the client. The issue of technical competence is usually defined in terms of one's education, training, and supervised experience in the area of practice. In contrast, specialization is defined by one's competence in a specialized area in which the specialist is considered more competent in the area of specialty than is the average general practitioner.

Not everyone can handle the rigorous requirements for working with dissociative patients or performing child custody evaluations. Knowing when to refer to another practitioner is as important as knowing when to treat. As Canter et al. (1994) point out, "Merely having an interest in a particular area does not necessarily qualify one to practice in that area" (p. 34). As a colleague once quoted to me during a training seminar, "Half of being smart is knowing what you're dumb at" (Doverspike, 2004c). This point can be illustrated by some simple examples. In my own practice, although I am board certified in neuropsychology, I routinely refer *child* neuropsychological evaluations to other neuropsychologists. Similarly, although I provide numerous consultations for memory testing, I never perform "recovered memories" testing. In psychotherapy, I may provide cognitive-behavioral therapy (McCullough, 2000), but not dialectical behavior therapy (Linehan, 1987a, 1987b). Remember the advice, "Know what you know, and know what you *don't* know."

As a general rule, ethical problems are less likely to arise when practicing within one's area of competence. However, an exception to this rule may apply to specialists who have become overly comfortable *within* their area of competence, such as the neuropsychologist who finds "a little brain dysfunction" in almost anyone, the eating disorders therapist to whom everyone looks "a little bulimic," the therapist who suspects sexual abuse in every child with a bruise, or the educational specialist who is eager to diagnose "ADD" (the popular acronym which has seemingly replaced careful examination of the diagnostic criteria for Attention-Deficit/Hyperactivity Disorder). To use an old diagnostic observation, "It's easier to see what you know than it is to know what you see." The ethical implication of this observation is that the careful and conscientious clinician is always alert to evidence that may not support his or her initial intuitive impressions. Good diagnosticians often develop their diagnostic hypotheses through intuition, but they test their hypotheses through deductive reasoning (Doverspike, 1999d; E. O. Othmer & S. C. Othmer, 1989).

Practicing *outside* an area of competence is an ethical breach that can be especially tempting in the practice of managed care. Many closed provider panels have few, if any, therapists in certain specialties. A client may get a provider's name from a website directory or "800" phone number with little or no understanding of the provider's scope of practice. In fact, most managed care companies give no information to their callers about a provider's professional degree or licensure. For example, an insured patient who calls his or her managed care company for a referral for psychological testing and psychotropic medication will usually be given the names of three providers in the geographic area or zip code specified by the caller, although none of these names is likely to be a psychiatrist and at least one of the names is likely to be a mental health professional who provides neither testing nor prescriptions. In other words, a potential client referred by a managed care company will know nothing of the provider's education, training, competence, or limitations. As a provider, if you do not know the limits of your competence, you will be overcome by them. Again, knowing when to refer is as important as knowing when to treat. One national survey revealed that almost 25% of professional psychologists reported that they had either "rarely" or "sometimes" provided services outside their areas of competence (Pope, Tabachnick, & Keith-Spiegel, 1987).

If you decide to practice in an area beyond the boundaries of your competence, it is especially important to obtain continuing education, ongoing supervision, and case consultation. Specific standards for education, training, and supervised experience are established for areas of practice in which it is recognized that specialized training and expertise are necessary to be competent. We are no longer a profession of generalists but a profession of specialists. Again, the ethical dimension is competence. Partly as a consequence of increasingly higher standards of care and more stringent definitions of professional competence, psychotherapists have become increasingly specialized. There is an increasing trend toward certification of proficiency in specialty areas of practice. For example, specialty training is required in assessment areas such as in the use of Anatomically Detailed Dolls and in treatment modalities such as Eye Movement Desensitization and Reprocessing (EMDR). Going from A to Z, other examples include Anger Management, Biofeedback, Child

Custody Evaluations, Dialectical Behavior Therapy, Executive Coaching, Forensic Examination, Guardianship Evaluations, Health Psychology, Imago Therapy, and so on through the rest of the alphabet.

For psychologists, there are many guidelines that define competence, including some of the following examples: "Guidelines for therapy with women" (APA Task Force on Sex Bias and Sex Role Stereotyping in Psychotherapeutic Practice, 1978), "Specialty Guidelines for Forensic Psychologists" (Committee on Ethical Guidelines for Forensic Psychologists, 1991), "Guidelines for providers of psychological services to ethnic, linguistic, and culturally diverse populations" (APA Office of Ethnic Minority Affairs, 1993), "Guidelines for child custody evaluations in divorce proceedings" (APA, 1994), "Guidelines for psychological evaluations in child protection matters" (APA Committee on Professional Practice and Standards, 1999), "Guidelines for psychotherapy with lesbian, gay, and bisexual clients" (APA Division 44/Committee on Lesbian, Gay, and Bisexual Concerns Task Force, 2000), "Guidelines for psychological practice with older adults" (APA Division 12 Section II and Division 20 Interdivisional Task Force on Practice of Clinical Geropsychology, 2003), "Guidelines for the evaluation of dementia and age-related cognitive decline" (APA Presidential Task Force on the Assessment of Age-Consistent Memory Decline and Dementia, 1998), and so on. Clinicians practicing in specialty areas for which recognized standards do not yet exist should take reasonable steps to ensure competence and to protect others from harm. Remember the adage, "Today's guidelines are tomorrow's standards of care."

The aforementioned discussion of competence focuses on *technical* competence, which is based on knowledge ("in your head") and skills ("with your hands"). There are two other types of competence that have received attention in the literature. These other types include intellectual competence and emotional competence. *Intellectual* competence refers to one's basic cognitive capacities, which are assumed to be intact in anyone capable of undergoing clinical training and capable of functioning as a mental health professional. Intellectual competence becomes of greater concern when a clinician is suspected of suffering from diminished capacity or cognitive impairment, which can be the result of a medical, neurological, or substance-related disorder. *Emotional* competence refers to one's emotional, psychological, and interpersonal functioning, which are also assumed to be intact in anyone capable of functioning as a mental health professional. Emotional competence becomes of greater concern when a clinician is suspected of suffering from an emotional or psychological disturbance, which can be the result of an adjustment reaction, relational problem, mental disorder, or a substance-related disorder. Emotional competence can also be associated with environmental stress, workaholic syndrome, and burnout syndrome (Freudenberger, 1980; Kilburn, Nathan, & Thoreson, 1986). Maintaining emotional competence requires cultivating vitality and creating a sense of balance in one's life through self-care. Borrowing from the Adlerian perspective, Myers, Sweeney, and Witmer (2000) identify five life tasks on their "wheel to wellness" that are a basic part of health functioning. These life tasks include spirituality, self-direction, work and leisure, friendship, and love. Paradoxically, it is often when one's resources are needed the most by others that one most significantly needs the renewal of those resources. In other words, renew your own resources first, because only then will you be able to give to others.

SUPERVISE ONLY
WHAT YOU KNOW

Practicing within one's area of competence is not only a concern for those undergoing supervision; it is a prerequisite for those *providing* supervision. Clinicians providing supervision to others need to be aware that supervision involves considerable responsibility and needs to be taken seriously. One rule of thumb is, "Do not supervise what you cannot do" (Bennett, Harris, & Remar, 1995, 1996, 1997; Harris, 2004; Younggren, 2006). Supervisors should also be "well trained, knowledgeable, and skilled in the practice of clinical supervision" (Stoltenberg & Delworth, 1987, p. 175). When there are unusual circumstances that require a supervisor to practice outside of the area of competence of his or her supervisor, it is the supervisor's responsibility to arrange for competent supervision (Cobia & Boes, 2000). As G. Corey et al. (2007) emphasize, "Supervisors are ultimately responsible, *both ethically and legally*, for the actions of their trainees" (p. 351).

Supervision involves at least twice as much professional liability as does psychotherapy. As Harris (2004) points out, "Every one of your supervisee's patients is your patient." The supervisor incurs both primary and secondary liability (Harrar, VandeCreek, & Knapp, 1990). Primary or direct liability relates to the supervisor's direct liability to the supervisee. Secondary liability, which is also known as indirect or vicarious liability, relates to the supervisor's vicarious liability to all of the clients of the supervisee. In other words, the supervisor is not only held ethically and legally responsible for the actions of the supervisee but the supervisor is also held responsible for the supervisee's clients.

Because supervisors assume the ultimate responsibility for all of their supervisees' actions, high-risk areas of practice require special consideration during supervision. Examples of high-risk situations include supervisee boundary violations with clients, treatment of life-endangering patients, and the use of memory retrieval techniques with adult survivors of childhood abuse (Knapp & VandeCreek, 1997). Koocher and Keith-Spiegel (1998) have pointed out that lack of timely feedback "is at the root of many ethical complaints that grow out of supervisory relationships" (p. 324). In a study of the quality of supervision in the counseling field, Ladany and colleagues (1999) found that 51% of 151 supervisees reported what they considered to be at least one ethical violation by their supervisors, with 33% of the supervisees reporting that they did not provide adequate evaluation of the supervisee's performance. Documentation of supervision sessions should reflect the quality of care given to the client as well as the quality of supervision provided to the supervisee (Bridge & Bascue, 1988; Knapp & VandeCreek, 1997).

OBTAIN ADEQUATE
INFORMED CONSENT

Informed consent has become an increasingly important concept as clinicians have become more aware of evolving ethical standards and relevant case law. In an age of litigation, it is important to remember that "psychologists can be held liable for failure to obtain appropriate informed consent *even if their subsequent treatment of the patient is exemplary from a clinical perspective*" (Stromberg & Dellinger, 1993, p. 5). In the practice of managed care, informed consent has become an even greater concern as case managers and utilization reviewers require disclosure of information that may result in a reduction of benefits or a limitation in the number of treatment sessions that are authorized. Although eventually beyond the clinician's control, submission of an insurance claim for payment of the treatment of a mental disorder can also have implications regarding the future insurability of a patient.

Ethical issues relevant to informed consent are addressed in the APA (2002) Ethical Standard 3.10(a), which in part states that, "When psychologists conduct research or provide assessment therapy, counseling, or consulting services in person or via electronic transmission or other forms of communication, they obtain the informed consent of the individual or individuals using language that is reasonably understandable to that person or persons except when conducting such activities without consent is mandated by law or governmental regulation or as otherwise provided in this Ethics Code" (p. 1065).*

Although the specific content of informed consent may differ in each situation, there are four basic elements that provide a foundation for understanding informed consent. Informed consent generally implies that (a) the person has competence, or the capacity to consent; (b) the person has been informed of significant information concerning the procedure; (c) the person has freely and voluntarily expressed consent without any undue influence; and (d) the consent process has been appropriately documented. In other words, the process of obtaining informed consent is not simply a matter of the client "signing off" on a series of forms. Instead, it is an ongoing process of communication that begins at the outset of treatment and continues as events unfold throughout the course of treatment.

The process of informed consent should involve ongoing communication, clarification, and decision making (Pope & Vasquez, 1991, 1998; Welfel, 2006). In keeping with the spirit of this process, clinicians have a duty to determine (informally or otherwise) whether the client is competent to give informed consent or whether the situation may justify rendering some type of service in the absence of fully informed consent. When a client is legally incapable of giving informed consent, the provider must obtain informed permission from a legally authorized person, such as parent or legal guardian, if such substitute consent is permitted by law. In addition, the provider has a duty to inform the client about the proposed interventions, seek the client's assent to those interventions, and consider the client's preferences and best interests. For a competent person who is fully capable of giving consent, the provider must consider whether the client has been provided with the relevant information to make an informed decision and whether the client sufficiently understands the information. As a final consideration, the provider must determine whether the client can provide consent on an adequately voluntary basis. Because treatment is an ongoing process, the client must adequately understand and voluntarily agree to any changes in the ongoing treatment plan. For example, informed consent considerations addressed during the 10th session of psychotherapy may be very different from those addressed during the initial interview. Haas and Malouf (2005) describe informed consent as a process, "perhaps

---

beginning with more general and global descriptions of the elements of treatment and later progressing to specific descriptions of specific procedures as needed" (pp. 61-62).

Informed consent considerations take on even greater significance with the use of more invasive or innovative procedures. From a risk-management perspective, it is interesting to note some of the changes that have taken place in the provisions of the *Psychologist's Professional Liability Insurance Policy* administered by the American Psychological Association Insurance Trust (APAIT). Although a special stipulation regarding the use of physical contact is no longer required, at one time APAIT-insured psychologists who offered services "involving physical contact with clients" were required to submit a written explanation including "the percent of clients receiving physical contact and a copy of the release form" (APAIT, 1996, p. 2). As a general rule, the more invasive or innovative the procedure, the greater the need for adequately informed consent and careful documentation of procedures (Doverspike, 1997b, 1999c). Because adequate informed consent procedures are so important in helping to prevent ethical problems before they arise, such procedures are discussed in greater detail later in this book in the chapter on Informed Consent (Chapter 2, pp. 25-44).

Whether one chooses a more casual question-answer format or a formal, written, narrative approach to obtaining informed consent, compliance with the APA ethical standard requires that the client's consent be "appropriately documented." Most proponents (Bennett et al., 1995, 1996, 1997, 2006; Harris, 2004; Harris & Remar, 1998; Schlosser & Tower, 1991; Younggren, 1995, 2006) advocate the use of a signed, detailed, and well-documented informed consent procedure. Consent forms should reflect, but should never replace, the ongoing dialogue between clinician and client. Those interested in an aspirational standard of care should consider the use of a combined verbal discussion and written documentation approach which "provides persuasive evidence that a conscientious effort to obtain informed consent was made" (Stromberg et al., 1988, p. 451).

BE AWARE OF CHILD CUSTODY EVALUATIONS

Although mentioned in an earlier section on practicing within one's area of competence, child custody evaluations stand apart from other areas because they are a major area in which ethics complaints are filed against psychologists. Over the past several years, state licensing boards have received an increasing number of complaints related to this litigious area (Younggren, 2006). In some states, custody evaluators can expect to have licensing board complaints or professional liability complaints routinely filed against them by noncustodial parents (Harris, 2004).

The greatest risks seem to occur with clinicians who do not have extensive training and experience in this area. Although a clinician may have good intentions, serious consequences can be caused by errors in judgment or by failing to be aware of the many pitfalls in performing custody evaluations (Ellis, 2006). For example, it would be considered unethical for a clinician to conduct a custody evaluation involving a couple or family with whom the clinician has a current or prior therapeutic or other conflicting relationship (Greenberg & Shuman, 1997; Morris, 1997). Although clients may be forgiving of the lapses on the part of a well-liked therapist, the same clients may not be forgiving of the lapses made by a therapist acting in the role of a custody evaluator who writes a report contrary to their interests. It is important to remember that the conflict that necessitates an independent custody determination usually does not involve one but two angry parents—which essentially doubles the liability risk for the evaluator. When opposing attorneys, expert witnesses, and the high stakes of "loss from evaluation" are added to the equation, the liability risk increases exponentially in comparison to other nonforensic areas of practice.

Because we live in a culture that "permits everything and forgives nothing" (Shapiro, 1994), clinicians who perform custody evaluations should be aware of the associated risks. Proficiency in conducting custody evaluations requires competence in several areas, including child development, psychological assessment, family system dynamics, and forensic testimony. Clinicians performing custody evaluations should be familiar with the "Guidelines for child custody evaluations in divorce proceedings" (APA, 1994). In addition to knowledge of professional standards, knowledge of the customary and usual professional practices is also important (M. J. Ackerman & M. C. Ackerman, 1997). Particularly when practicing in a high-risk specialty area involving litigation, the usual and customary risk-management considerations (such as obtaining informed consent and documenting one's decisions in writing) take on even greater significance.

MAINTAIN CLEAR
BOUNDARIES WITH CLIENTS

A colleague on a state license board once said that the single best way to avoid the most serious of ethics complaints was to "never have sex with a client." One might add, "or a former client." This advice may seem so obvious that it doesn't need repeating, yet this issue concerns the most serious ethical breach of our profession. Indeed, having sex with a client is generally considered the most egregious unethical behavior, regardless of one's professional identity or theoretical orientation (Borys & Pope, 1989). Sexual impropriety accounts for approximately half of the costs of malpractice cases and over 20% of the total number of claims (Pope, 1989a; Pope & Vasquez, 1991; Stromberg & Dellinger, 1993). Increasingly, in an effort to reduce such claims, professional liability insurance policies have excluded coverage of sexual impropriety. Even when allegations of sexual impropriety cannot be proved, such cases often involve multiple nonsexual violations that can readily be substantiated.

Sexual misconduct was one of the most frequent reasons for disciplinary actions for psychologists from 1983 to 2001 (K. Kirkland, K. L. Kirkland, & Reaves, 2004). Although many studies have focused on psychologists, the only national study using the same survey instrument during the same time period with respondents from three major mental health professions found *no significant difference* among the rates at which psychiatrists, psychologists, and social workers acknowledged engaging in sex with their patients (Borys & Pope, 1989). Borys and Pope reported that 0.5% of their respondents acknowledged having engaged in sexual activity with a current client, and 3.9% of the respondents acknowledged having engaged in sexual activity with a client after termination.

Gabbard and Pope (1988) have documented the many harmful effects of "professional incest." In almost every complaint of sexual misconduct there are also other boundary violations as well. Even when allegations of sexual misconduct cannot be proved, allegations of other boundary violations can almost always be proved. When boundary violations begin to occur, a clinician may start sliding down the slippery slope toward sexual misconduct. Although a mandatory ethical obligation would be to "never have sex with a client," a more aspirational standard would be to "maintain clear boundaries with clients." By way of analogy, everyone knows that a driver shouldn't fall asleep at the wheel while driving. Although some people do fall asleep, the warning line should not be "don't fall asleep at the wheel," but rather "don't drive when you are tired."

Good boundaries begin with driving on the right side of the road. Occasionally, there may be a reason to cross the white center line, which like any boundary crossing requires caution and careful consideration. However, it is not reasonable to cross the solid yellow line, which like any boundary violation means that there is a chance of harm. If good driving depends on boundaries, then good relationships certainly depend on good boundaries. Whether sitting in the driver's seat or in the psychotherapist's chair, remember to maintain clear boundaries.

USE PROJECTIVE RETROSPECTIVE THINKING

Before you take action in a situation, try to *anticipate* the possible consequences of your actions and *think* how your actions will be viewed later if you have to explain them to a respected colleague. In cognitive-behavioral psychotherapy, this strategy is known as "consequential thinking." In addictive disease relapse prevention (Marlatt, 1985), it is called "thinking the drink through." In professional liability risk management, it is called "projective retrospective" thinking (Bennett et al., 1996; E. Harris, personal communication, April 22, 1996).

Eric Harris (personal communication, April 22, 1996) coined the term "projective retrospective" thinking to refer to consequential thinking in which one anticipates the future consequences of one's actions. When one is contemplating taking an action in a particular situation, one is advised to think forward (projectively) and then look back (retrospectively) on one's anticipated actions with respect to their possible consequences (Harris & Remar, 1998). The concept of "projective retrospective" thinking is a recurrent theme in annual risk-management seminars sponsored by the American Psychological Association Insurance Trust (APAIT; Bennett et al., 1995, 1996, 1997; Harris, 2004; Younggren, 2006).

A colleague once jokingly told me, "If you can't explain it to your mother, you shouldn't be doing it." Another good rule of thumb would be, "If you can't explain it to your licensing board, you shouldn't be doing it." In other words, use projective retrospective thinking. Project yourself into the future, and then think how you would look back on your actions if you were to be retrospectively evaluated. Even better, when writing your progress notes, think how your actions will later look to someone reading them. Think how your actions will sound to your client's attorney in court. If you think your rationale and decisions sound good to you in your office, think how they will sound to others if you have to explain them in court.

CONSULT WITH A COLLEAGUE

From time to time, everyone faces situations that require special consideration beyond one's own best judgment. The smart counselor learns from his or her mistakes, but the wise counselor learns from the mistakes of others. The wise counselor also knows when to identify those situations that deserve consultation with a peer. Peer consultation means talking with a respected colleague who is impartial, objective, and knowledgeable. It does *not* mean talking to someone who will simply agree with whatever actions you have already taken. A good peer is someone who can help you see your ethical blind spots.

If you are not sure whom to call, one option is to call your most respected colleague. To avoid unintentional self-interest, make sure he or she is a colleague who can give you an objective opinion that is not clouded by your relationship. A second option, which offers a more objective "arms-length" consultation, is to call your local professional association and request an ethics consultation. A third option is to call the ethics consultant or legal counsel of your professional liability insurance company. Two heads are usually better than one; a brief consultation is better than none.

Good motives can sometimes lead to bad results. Sooner or later, everyone faces a situation in which one's best efforts may result in adverse consequences. In such situations, the best defense is to have obtained and documented peer consultation. Such documentation will at least demonstrate careful consideration of appropriate standards of care. Peer consultations are particularly important when clinicians are faced with situations in which the clinician must consider actions in high-risk situations (e.g., dispensing with informed consent, involuntarily committing a suicidal client, breaching confidentiality in a duty-to-protect situation, performing child custody evaluations, terminating psycho-therapy with a noncompliant client, and so forth).

Although there are some ethicists who advise clinicians to "consult on every case" (Pope, 1989b), this strategy can be difficult at best. If you *don't* consult on every single case, there is another strategy that can sometimes help: Visualize your most respected colleague sitting in the consultation room with you and your client. While picturing your colleague in front of you, think to yourself, "What would he or she do? What would he or she say?" If you're *still* not sure, you should definitely consult with a peer.

DOCUMENT YOUR
DECISIONS IN WRITING

Remember the old documentation rule, "If it wasn't written, it wasn't done." It is not only important to document what you *did*; it is also important to document what you *didn't* do (Harris, 2004; Stromberg et al., 1988). Get in the habit of making contemporaneous notes, including time and date of entry. In retrospective review, your notes are your best (and sometimes only) evidence that you have been a careful and conscientious clinician. In situations involving unfounded complaints, a well-documented record is always the best defense. A psychologist who had been investigated by a state licensing board once called me to express his frustration with the absence of due process in which the investigator would not reveal the name of the complainant or the specific nature of the complaint. The psychologist lived in a state in which the licensing board was not required to inform the psychologist of the specific nature of the complaint. I suggested that the psychologist consult with an attorney, request from the state board the name of the person who had filed the complaint, and then obtain the client's permission to release the complete clinical record to the licensing board. Several months later, after the licensing board had closed the case as frivolous, I asked the psychologist how he had managed to defend himself against a complaint that was never revealed to him. He simply smiled and said, "I just gave them my notes, and I had *lots* of notes."

Whenever I have obtained legal consultations, there is one bit of advice I always hear: "Put it in writing." Adequate record keeping provides the first indication to attorneys that a practitioner's treatment meets minimum standards of care. I have gotten to the point where I not only "put it in writing," but I often imagine the client's attorney reading my notes as I write them. It has been suggested that clinicians "hallucinate on their shoulder the image of a hostile prosecuting attorney who might preside at the trial in which their records are subpoenaed" (Gutheil, 1980, p. 481). In discussing the client record as a tool in risk management, Piazza and Yeager (1991) recommend that psychologists "not write anything in the client's records that you would not want a client's lawyer to read" (p. 344). As a general rule, write your notes the way you would like to read them in court. Even better, as one hospital attorney has advised, "Write your notes the way you would like someone *else* to read them in court" (J. D. Doverspike, personal communication, November 1, 1996).

Gutheil (1980, p. 479) suggests that clinicians "use paranoia as a motivating force" in writing progress notes and keeping effective records for forensic purposes, utilization review, and good treatment planning. Although minimum requirements for record keeping are contained in statutory law and various accreditation guidelines, there are no maximum standards for record keeping. In other words, "There is a floor, but no ceiling, on what to write" (Gutheil, 1980, p. 480). The "General Guidelines for Providers of Psychological Services" (APA, 1987) contains the recommendation that case notes minimally include dates and types of services as well as any "significant actions taken" (p. 717). Ideally, notes should also include a summary of topics discussed, techniques or interventions employed during the session, and the client's reaction. In order to minimize subjectivity or unsupported impressions, any clinical inferences or interpretations should be supported by behavioral observations. One useful sentence structure involves the following format: "Client appeared [clinical interpretation], as evidenced by [behavioral observation]."

On a more aspirational level of record keeping, for each significant client-therapist treatment decision, the record should include (a) what the choice is expected to accomplish, (b) why the clinician believes it will be effective, (c) any risks that might be involved and why they are justified, (d) what alternative treatments were considered, (e) why they were rejected, and (f) what steps were taken to improve the effectiveness of chosen treatment (Soisson, VandeCreek, & Knapp, 1987). In other words, document what you did and why you did it, but also document what you didn't do and why you didn't do it (Stromberg et al., 1988). Gutheil (1980, p. 482) recommends that the clinician "think out loud in the record" so that one's notes reflect active concern for the client's welfare and consideration of various interventions. Gutheil emphasizes, "As a general rule, the more uncertainty there is, the more one should think out loud in the record" (p. 482). In summary, "Write your progress notes in a user-friendly way so they can be read by your client in your office, and write them in a risk-managed way so they can be read by your client's attorney in court" (Doverspike, 2006b, p. 14).

KEEP COMMUNICATION
CHANNELS OPEN

In the practice of medicine, it has often been said that one of the best ways to avoid a malpractice lawsuit is to maintain open communication while treating the patient with kindness and respect. Mistakes happen and people are usually more forgiving when their doctor has had an ongoing open and honest relationship with them. Kovacs (1984) makes the observation that, "Those who are involved in meaningful dialogues are not likely to sue each other" (p. 12). A recurring theme at the APAIT risk-management workshops is that good communication is associated with reduced professional liability claims (Younggren, 2006). These words of wisdom are supported by empirical evidence, as illustrated in the studies cited below.

A study funded by the Agency for Health Care Policy and Research (AHCPR) reveals that primary care physicians who listen to their patients and use a friendlier manner during visits may reduce their risk of being sued for malpractice (*Good Communication Is a Key Factor in Avoiding Malpractice Suits*, 1997). In this AHCPR study, Levinson and colleagues (1997) found that primary care physicians in a "no claims" group spent more time with patients (an average of 18.3 minutes vs. 15.0 minutes) during a routine office visit than physicians in the "claims group." In addition to length of the visit, physicians in the "no claims group" were more likely to tell patients what was going to happen during the office visit by using phrases like, "First I'm going to examine you and then we will talk the problem over." Physicians who had no malpractice claims filed against them also asked patients for their opinions, elicited questions from patients, and were more likely to laugh and use humor during an office visit. Levinson, Gorawara-Bhat, and Lamb (2000) linked good communication with fewer professional liability claims. Hickson et al. (2002) linked communication lapses and patient complaints to professional liability claims. When a patient complaint or dissatisfaction is coupled with an adverse event, the patient is more likely to sue the physician when the physician has not satisfactorily addressed the patient's complaint.

In the early years of my hospital practice, I once witnessed a "shotgun" malpractice suit in which several physicians were named in the lawsuit yet one physician was unexpectedly excluded from the ordeal (Doverspike, 1997c, 1999c). The patient later disclosed to me that the one physician who was spared had done his best to treat her with respect and keep communication channels open during a difficult involuntary hospitalization. Similarly, I have known both psychologists and psychiatrists whose communication skills have allowed them to identify and resolve major patient dissatisfactions before those rose to the level of formal complaints. On the other hand, I have also had patients tell me that they had filed complaints against their physicians because "my doctor never talked to me" or, more often, "My doctor never *listened.*" In listening to these stories and in consulting with physicians over the years, I have been reminded repeatedly how important it is to keep communication channels open. Remember the adage, "Psychologists are doctors who listen."

A forensic psychologist once estimated that 95% of malpractice complaints could be prevented by "treating your patient with respect and kindness and as a person from whom you can learn a great deal" (Sutton, 1986). In my own experience, I have found that conflicts with clients can usually be minimized or avoided altogether by discussing concerns at the outset. When conflicts do arise, discussing the issue first is usually the best path toward successful resolution. I am often surprised by the number of clients who say that they had not discussed their concerns with their respective therapists before filing a complaint. Client dissatisfactions that are addressed at the source rarely rise to the level of formal complaints. Because mental health professionals are in the business of communicating with others, it makes sense to use communication as a cornerstone of ethical practice management.

According to attorneys James W. Saxton and Maggie M. Finkelstein, "Often times, anger drives a patient to a plaintiff's attorney." In their article on using good communication and providing "five star service" to reduce malpractice liability risk, Saxton and Finkelstein (2005) provide a rationale for handling patient complaints:

> The complaints should be looked upon as an opportunity: to address a patient concern, to prevent the concern from escalating, to create evidence in your own favor should the matter evolve, to satisfy a patient, and to prevent the same situation from occurring again either to the same patient or any other patient as part of an overall quality improvement program. (p. 3)

Remember that there is no such thing as a frivolous complaint. Given the amount of time and the enormous emotional (and often financial) resources required to resolve formal complaints, it is important to take all client dissatisfactions seriously. A good working relationship with your client may help guarantee that your client will report dissatisfactions directly to *you* rather than to someone else. In the event that your client makes a complaint directly to you, the best course of action would be to take the complaint seriously, discuss the client's concerns, work toward a satisfactory resolution, obtain consultation with a peer, and document your actions in writing. Of course, the exception to this rule would apply in the unfortunate event that a lawsuit happens to arise, in which case the clinician would be advised to cease communicating with the client and begin consulting with an attorney (Bennett et al., 1990; Harris, 2004; Younggren, 2006).

ASPIRE TO A STANDARD
OF EXCELLENCE

Mark Twain (1901) once said, "Always do right. This will gratify some people, and astonish the rest." This wisdom reflects an important risk-management strategy for ethical responsibility. Ethical temptations are not an indication of weakness but of strength. As conscientious practitioners, we are not tempted to do what we cannot do but rather what is within our ability to do. In other words, the greater the ability, the greater the temptation. At the same time, the greater the ability, the greater the aspiration to a standard of excellence. To whom much is given in the way of knowledge, much is due in the way of responsibility. The ethically responsible practitioner avoids ethical pitfalls by striving for ethical excellence.

In discussing the characteristics of the ethically responsible professional, Van Hoose and Paradise (1979) suggest that a counselor "is probably acting in an ethically responsible way concerning a client if (1) he or she has maintained personal and professional honesty, coupled with (2) the best interests of the client, (3) without malice or personal gain, and (4) can justify his or her actions as the best judgment of what should be done based upon the current state of the profession" (p. 58).

Psychologists interested in an aspirational level of ethical awareness might be interested in reviewing literature such as *Ethics for Psychologists: A Commentary on the APA Ethics Code* (Canter et al., 1994) and *Ethical Conflicts in Psychology* (Bersoff, 2003), which contain practical case discussions, empirical research, and scholarly commentaries related to various ethics topics. Counselors interested in achieving excellence in ethical aspirations might be interested in reviewing the *American Counseling Association Ethical Standards Casebook* (Herlihy & G. Corey, 2006).

AN ALTERNATIVE VIEW:
THE MYTH OF RISK MANAGEMENT

No discussion of ethical risk management would be complete without considering an alternative point of view. Although my own position is a relatively conservative risk-managed approach, I am indebted to my colleague Ofer Zur for raising my consciousness by challenging orthodox ethical dogma and offering alternative perspectives that promote meaningful discussion of the complex issues involved in dual relationships and psychotherapy. There are at least three counterpoint views to the prevailing conventional wisdom of risk management. One hypothesis, which has been referred to as the *curse of risk management*, maintains the position that risk-managed strategies do not even lower the risk of ethical complaints or lawsuits in the first place. A second hypothesis, which has been referred to as the *myth of risk management*, maintains that we as mental health professionals have brought the problem of increased ethical complaints and malpractice lawsuits on ourselves through our continued efforts at raising the bar of the standard of care. A third hypothesis, which might be referred to as the *worst of risk management*, states that by being motivated by a fear of lawsuits rather than by a compassion for clients, mental health professionals actually commit the worst of all ethical violations. Each of these perspectives is briefly addressed below.

The Curse of
Risk Management

One of the most noticeable trends in the field of professional ethics has been the continued use of ethics codes to establish standards of care in professional liability suits and in the adjudication of complaints by state licensing boards. Over the last decade, the standard of care has been raised not only by expert witnesses for plaintiffs, but also by expert speakers at professional liability risk-management seminars. Although the goal of ethical and legal risk-management seminars has been to reduce malpractice complaints, one unintended consequence of the risk-management movement has been an increase in "continuingly raising the bar as to what constitutes acceptable practice" (Williams, 2003, p. 203). As one psychologist and attorney observed the situation, "Well-intentioned efforts to reduce the risk of litigation have, in fact, increased the risks to which professionals are exposed" (Fleer, 1999, p. 57). As a result, one of the ironies of risk management is that mental health professionals themselves may have unwittingly contributed to an "increase, rather than a decrease, [in] complaints to licensing boards and lawsuits in civil courts" (Williams, 2003, p. 203). Recent revisions of professional ethics codes have attempted to reverse this trend. For example, because the 1992 APA Ethics Code was often used by trial lawyers and expert witnesses to define the standard of care in malpractice litigation, the writers of the 2002 APA Ethics Code inserted protective language in the form of a specific disclaimer that states, "The Ethics Code is *not* [italics added] intended to be a basis of civil liability" (2002, p. 1061).

In his article titled "The curse of risk management," Martin Williams (2003) notes that the paradoxical effect of increasing the numbers of ethics complaints and liability suits occurs for two reasons. First, over a period of time, restrictions that were once merely risk management suggestions eventually evolve to become the perceived standard of care. The prototypic risk-managed recommendation is discussed so much among colleagues that it essentially becomes accepted as the prevailing standard of care. In other words, today's guidelines become tomorrow's standards of care. As Williams puts it, "If enough practitioners believe that a standard exists, then, for all practical purposes, it does exist" (p. 204). Second, practitioners, as well as expert witnesses who testify against practitioners on behalf of civil plaintiffs and licensing boards, tend to confuse risk management with standard of care. Something that once seemed like a good risk-management suggestion shows up in expert testimony as if it were the readily accepted, agreed-upon standard of care. When a malpractice plaintiff has to prove a breach of a standard of care, all it takes to establish the standard of care is the opinion of the expert witnesses. In other words, it is your expert against mine.

The Myth of Risk Management

The risk-managed approach itself is not without its critics. At least some of the criticism is based on the assumption that practitioners may be utilizing risk-management strategies that are not necessarily needed in the first place. This hypothesis maintains that although such strategies may reduce anxiety on the part of the practitioner, these strategies do not necessarily reduce malpractice because it is such a low frequency behavior in the first place.

Despite the furor over malpractice tort reform, a survey by Studdert et al. (2006) finds no support for the widespread belief that the medical profession is stricken with frivolous litigation. The authors studied a random sample of 1,452 closed malpractice claims from five insurers in four areas of the country and concluded that the tort system works reasonably well in separating claims without merit from those with merit and compensating the latter. Studdert et al. state, "the profile of non-error claims we observed does not square with the notion of opportunistic trial lawyers pursuing questionable lawsuits" (p. 2030).

In what might be described as the myth of risk management, it has been noted that the absolute frequency of malpractice complaints is so low statistically that such suits would usually not occur even in the absence of risk-managed recommendations (Williams, 2003, p. 202). In other words, the low base rate of malpractice suits makes it difficult to determine which, if any, set of behaviors actually reduces the statistical probability of such suits. From an operant behavioral perspective, it is as if the risk-managed strategies are superstitious behaviors maintained by the presence of intermittent reinforcement (i.e., anxiety reduction) in the absence of aversive outcomes.

The Worst of Risk Management

Perhaps the best critique of risk management comes from Lazarus (2002) who says, "If I am to summarize my position in one sentence, I would say that one of the worst professional or ethical violations is that of permitting current risk-management principles to take precedence over humane interventions" (p. 31). Similarly, if I am to summarize my own position in one sentence, I would state, "Reasonable clinicians protect themselves by protecting their patients" (Doverspike, 2004a, p. 210), and one of the best ways to protect the patient is to aspire to excellence in providing a reasonable standard of care.

SUMMARY OF ETHICAL RISK-MANAGEMENT CONSIDERATIONS

As a member of a state ethics committee, I have personally observed that ethics committees often spend hours upon hours deliberating the merits of complaints that could have been avoided altogether had the clinician simply spent 15 minutes consulting with a colleague in the first place (Doverspike, 1997c). In situations involving unfounded complaints, a well-documented record is always the best defense. A clinician's best ethical risk-management strategy includes understanding relevant ethical and legal principles, utilizing an ethical decision-making plan, obtaining adequate informed consent, practicing within an area of competence, treating the client with respect and kindness, keeping communication channels open, obtaining peer consultation on a regular basis, and documenting the record as if the client's attorney were reading it. As a general rule of thumb, it is easier to avoid a complaint than it is to defend one. Remember the advice, "Prevention is better than intervention" (C. Webb, personal communication, June 4, 2004). At the same time, the risk-management approach is not without its critics. Fear of lawyers should never replace compassion for clients as a motivating force. Reasonable practitioners protect themselves by protecting their patients, and one of the best ways of protecting patients is to practice a reasonable standard of care.

POINTS TO REMEMBER

- Understand ethical and legal standards. When in doubt, read the manual.
- Always obtain adequately informed consent.
- Practice within your area of competence.
- Beware of child custody evaluations.
- Maintain clear boundaries with clients and former clients.
- Use "projective retrospective" or consequential thinking.
- Consult with a colleague. Two heads are better than one.
- Document your decisions in writing.
- Keep communication channels open with your client.
- Aspire to a standard of ethical excellence.
- Remember it is easier to avoid a complaint than it is to defend one.
- Protect yourself by protecting your patient.

Chapter Two

Informed Consent Considerations: Preventing Ethical Problems Before They Arise

In an article on the topic of how to avoid malpractice, Barnett (1997) shares the observation, "Too often I have experienced that sinking feeling in the pit of my stomach when reviewing an ethics complaint, seeing how costly this is to the individuals involved and often how easily it could have been avoided" (p. 20). When listening to deliberations in ethics committee meetings, I also often experience that sinking feeling in the pit of my stomach when I realize how easily an ethics problem could have been avoided in the first place by anticipating and preventing the problem in advance through the use of a process of adequate informed consent. Whereas ethical decision-making models provide a *reactive* approach to solving ethical problems, the process of informed consent may be viewed as a *proactive* approach to preventing ethical problems before they arise.

Informed consent has become an increasingly important concept as clinicians have become more aware of evolving ethical standards and relevant case law. Informed consent has become a popular topic in continuing education and risk-management training (Bennett et al., 1995, 1996; Harris, 2004; Shapiro, 1994; R. Smith et al., 1994; Younggren, 2005, 2006). Although questions have been raised about whether informed consent procedures provide any protection against legal liability, there is no question that *failure* to obtain informed consent is a proven area of legal risk (Stromberg & Dellinger, 1993; Weiner & Wettstein, 1993). The first landmark legal case involving informed consent in the field of medicine was *Canterbury v. Spence* (1972), which defined the elements of modern informed consent and the need for full disclosure of the possible effects of a therapeutic procedure. Based on what is known as the "patient criterion," the ruling in *Canterbury v. Spence* defined full disclosure as "what the typical patient would want to know." In an age of increasing litigation, "psychologists can be held liable for failure to obtain appropriate informed consent *even if their subsequent treatment of the patient is exemplary from a clinical perspective*" (Stromberg & Dellinger, 1993, p. 5). In the practice of managed care, informed consent has become a concern to providers as utilization reviewers request confidential information necessary to establish medical necessity, evaluate treatment outcome, and limit services rendered to patients. Because a history of having received treatment for a mental disorder can have implications regarding the future insurability of a patient, the seemingly simple act of submitting an insurance claim can have implications that underscore the importance of obtaining adequate informed consent.

At a time when client satisfaction questionnaires seem to be more popular than psychotherapy outcome studies, informed consent procedures may also make sense from a marketing perspective. An empirical investigation by Sullivan, Martin, and Handelsman (1993) found that a hypothetical male therapist was rated more highly if he used a consent form to promote discussion than an identical therapist who did not use an informed consent procedure. The authors concluded that the use of an informed consent procedure "seems to enhance impressions of trustworthiness and expertness" (p. 162). From an ethical perspective, Handelsman and Galvin (1988) have observed that written consent forms also "have a role in facilitating the ethical goals of informed consent: increasing professionals' self-scrutiny, respecting the autonomy of clients, and allowing clients to enhance their welfare by becoming partners with the therapist in their mental health care" (p. 223).

AN OVERVIEW OF
INFORMED CONSENT

What is the first thing that should be discussed with a client as part of the initial intake interview? The answer is *informed consent* considerations. Informed consent can be loosely defined as an agreement that ensures that the client's participation in treatment is voluntary and based on an understanding of the procedures and their related benefits, risks, and alternatives. In the field of medicine, Switankowsky (1998) proposes an autonomy-enhancing model of informed consent in which the patient-physician relationship is viewed as an equal partnership with a common goal of improving the client's overall health and well-being.

In the field of psychotherapy, Pope and Vasquez (1998) describe informed consent as a dynamic process that involves communication, clarification, and decision making. As the treatment plan changes, so does the ongoing requirement for informed consent. In keeping with the spirit of an ongoing, dynamic process, Handelsman and Galvin (1988) have developed an outline of questions that can be addressed as part of an informed consent discussion. Designed to facilitate discussion, their outline format includes questions related to outpatient therapy, appointments, confidentiality, and money. In emphasizing the advantages of their question-answer format over narrative forms, Handelsman and Galvin (1988) point out that their question-answer approach may be less overwhelming than a lengthy written form, and the conversational style of their format preserves the clients' right to *refuse* information. Of course, one could argue that a client's refusal of information could itself later prove problematic. Therapists should think twice before working with clients who don't agree with the therapist's policies (Harris, 2004). Most proponents (G. Corey et al., 2007; Haas & Malouf, 2005; Harris, 2004; Younggren, 2006) advocate the use of a signed, detailed, and well-documented informed consent procedure.

UNDERSTAND THE
ETHICAL PRINCIPLES

Ethical issues relevant to informed consent are addressed in APA (2002) Ethical Standard 10.01(a) (Informed Consent to Therapy) which in part states, "When obtaining informed consent to therapy as required in Standard 3.10, Informed Consent, psychologists inform clients/patients as early as is feasible in the therapeutic relationship about the nature and anticipated course of therapy, fees, involvement of third parties, and limits of confidentiality and provide sufficient opportunity for the client/patient to ask questions and receive answers" (p. 1072). Although the specific content of informed consent may differ in each situation, there are some basic elements that provide a foundation for understanding the ethical requirements of informed consent. With respect to these basic elements, it may be helpful to distinguish among the related concepts of notice, disclosure, assent, and consent. Although the terms *notice* and *disclosure* are often used interchangeably, they sometimes have a different connotation. *Notice* refers to information that is simply posted or provided in writing to all clients, such as a Patient's Bill of Rights or a Health Insurance Portability and Accountability Act (HIPAA, 1996) Privacy Notice that is posted on a wall, whereas *disclosure* is information that is personally disclosed to a client, such as the more specific nuances of information that are discussed with a client. In the practice of psychotherapy, a notice may be something as simple as a "Do not disturb" sign hung from a doorknob, while disclosure generally refers to information discussed with the client. *Assent* means that the client's continued cooperation and participation implies agreement with the procedures, whereas *consent* refers to the more formal process in which the client agrees to participate after being provided with significant information (made by disclosure of the therapist). Assent is generally implied by a client's continued cooperation, whereas consent is made explicit by verbal agreement.

APA Ethical Standards generally imply four elements of informed consent. Although the specific content of informed consent may differ in each situation, there are four basic elements that provide a foundation for understanding informed consent. Informed consent generally implies that the person (a) has competence, or the capacity to consent, (b) has been informed of significant information concerning the procedure, (c) has freely and voluntarily expressed consent without any undue influence, and that (d) the consent process has been appropriately documented. In other words, the process of obtaining informed consent is not simply a matter of the client "signing off" on consent forms. These four basic components of informed consent overlap with the medico-legal model described in *The Psychologist's Legal Handbook* (Stromberg et al., 1988). Stromberg et al. delineate the four components as "(1) *competency* of the patient, (2) disclosure of *material information*, (3) *understanding* by the patient, and (4) *voluntary consent*" (p. 447). Each of these components is discussed in more detail below.

DETERMINE
CAPACITY TO CONSENT

The first element of informed consent involves the issue of competence or "capacity to consent," which means that the client possesses "a basic ability rationally to assess the risks and benefits of treatment" (Stromberg & Dellinger, 1993, p. 5). For informed consent purposes, the issue of competency "means essentially that the person is able to understand the basic purposes and effects (including risks or side effects) of the proposed diagnostic procedure, therapy, or hospitalization" (Stromberg et al., 1988, p. 448). The psychologist has a duty to determine (informally or otherwise) whether the client is competent to give consent or whether the situation may justify providing some type of service in the absence of fully informed consent. The client's capacity to consent does not require formal documentation but rather must be based on the psychologist's *understanding* of the client at the time the consent is given (Canter et al., 1994).

When a client is legally incapable of giving informed consent, APA Ethical Standard 3.10(b) requires that "psychologists . . . obtain appropriate permission from a legally authorized person, if such substitute consent is permitted or required by law" (2002, p. 1065). In addition, the psychologist must inform the client about the proposed interventions, seek the client's assent to those interventions, and consider the client's preferences and best interests. Consultation with a colleague is also advisable in situations in which the client is unable to give consent (Canter et al., 1994). In cases involving children, the APA Ethical Standard does not require that the psychologist necessarily obtain the child's agreement, but simply that the psychologist explain the procedures, seek the child's assent, and consider the child's preferences and best interests (Canter et al., 1994). In the case of involuntarily hospitalized inpatients, under almost all state laws, involuntary commitment does not itself imply incompetence (Remar & Hubert, 1996; Stromberg & Dellinger, 1993). A more difficult situation arises in situations in which there is some question concerning the client's capacity to consent. In such cases, the psychologist is advised to engage the client in discussion, elicit input from others, and document how the client's rights have been considered and protected (Canter et al., 1994). As Haas and Malouf (2005) advise clinicians, "Assume that the person is competent to give informed consent unless there is clear evidence to the contrary" (p. 67).

PROVIDE SIGNIFICANT
INFORMATION

For a competent person who is fully capable of giving consent, the second basic element of informed consent requires that the person be informed of "significant information" regarding procedures. It is this second element of informed consent that has received the most attention from legal analysts and professional writers (Bennett et al., 1995, 1996; Shapiro, 1994; Stromberg & Dellinger, 1993; Weiner & Wettstein, 1993; Younggren, 1995). Stromberg et al. (1988) point out that courts have focused most closely on the client's *understanding*, even though it constitutes only one component of competency to give informed consent. The clinician must provide relevant information and determine whether the person sufficiently *understands* the information necessary to make an informed decision. This provision does not require that any *specific* type of information be provided, but rather that the client be provided with "significant information." Such information might include issues related to confidentiality, benefits and risks of treatment, and alternative forms of treatment.

Piazza and Baruth (1990) recommend that the psychologist furnish information related to the treatment to be provided, as well as its potential benefits and limitations. Stromberg et al. (1988) state, "The practitioner must disclose all information that a reasonable person would want to consider before deciding to accept or reject treatment, including the nature of treatment, its potential benefits and risks, the existence of any alternative treatments, its benefits and risks, and the benefits and risks of no treatment at all" (p. 449). Haas and Malouf (2005) offer some practical guidelines including, "Put yourself in the client's place; what information would *you* desire?" (p. 67). Remember the Golden Rule of informed consent: "Treat your client as you would want to be treated." In other words, provide your client with the same information that you would want provided to you. The important role of informed consent is to manage client expectations by creating reasonable expectations in the first place.

At a minimum, APA (2002) Ethical Standard 10.01(a) requires that psychologists provide significant information about "the nature and anticipated course of therapy, fees, involvement of third parties, and limits of confidentiality and provide sufficient opportunity for the client/patient to ask questions and receive answers" (p. 1072). Other relevant sections of the APA Ethical Standards also include fees and financial arrangements, couple and family relationships, use of assessments, discussing the limits of confidentiality, and providing therapy to those served by others.

The material contained on the CD-ROM that accompanies this book addresses many vital issues related to practice including consent forms, alternate procedures, limits of confidentiality, financial arrangements, and much, much more. A detailed list of that material can be found on pages xiii-xxii.

With respect to structuring therapy relationships, APA (2002) Ethical Standard 10.01(a) (Informed Consent to Therapy) "psychologists inform clients/patients as early as is feasible in the therapeutic relationship about the nature and anticipated course of therapy, fees, involvement of third parties, and limits of confidentiality and provide sufficient opportunity for the client/patient to ask questions and receive answers" (p. 1072). Further clarification of this standard may be derived with reference to the earlier APA (1992) Ethical Standard 4.01 (Structuring the Relationship), which states, "Psychologists make reasonable efforts to answer patients' questions and to avoid misunderstandings about therapy. Whenever possible, psychologists provide oral and/or written information, using language that is reasonably understandable to the patient or client" (1992, p. 1605). The question-answer approach advocated by Handelsman and Galvin (1988) certainly conforms to this standard. Regarding treatment information to be provided, Piazza and Baruth (1990) recommend that the psychologist discuss potential benefits and limitations of treatment. With respect to the issue of confidentiality, psychologists have traditionally been trained to inform their clients that their communications are confidential. However, contemporary psychologists are increasingly encouraged to emphasize the *exceptions* to confidentiality (Bennett et al., 1995, 1996; Shapiro, 1994; Younggren, 1995, 2006). For example, some practitioners provide the client with a list of some of the most common exceptions to confidentiality and inform the client that this may not be a comprehensive list.

What is the first thing that should be discussed with a client during the informed consent portion of the initial intake interview? The answer is not only confidentiality, but also, more importantly, the *exceptions* to confidentiality. Although exceptions to confidentiality are defined somewhat differently by the ethics codes of different professions and state licensing boards, there are some standard limits that are common to most professional ethics codes. These exceptions to confidentiality can be roughly divided into (a) *mandatory* disclosures, such as mandated reporting of suspected abuse of minors, elderly, and the disabled; (b) *discretionary* disclosures, such as reporting of imminent and foreseeable danger to the client or others, particularly in cases in which the client has made a threat against a readily identifiable person; and (c) *optional* or negotiated disclosures, such as reporting that is directed by the client, including submitting information to an insurance company, releasing information to a third party, and so forth. In couples and family therapy, optional or negotiated disclosures include those exceptions of confidentiality that are mutually agreed upon in advance by all parties (e.g., how the therapist will handle disclosures made privately to the therapist by one client). In child and adolescent therapy, optional or negotiated disclosures include those mutually agreed-upon circumstances in which confidential information about the minor child will be shared with the parents.

Although state laws may preempt federal HIPAA guidelines in cases in which state laws provide the patient greater protection of privacy or increased access to his or her records, there are some generally accepted exceptions to confidentiality contained in HIPAA regulations. These exceptions include (a) reasonable suspicions of the abuse or neglect of minor children, disabled and vulnerable adults, and the elderly (usually defined over age 65); (b) health oversight activities, such as the disclosure of protected health information by a licensed therapist in response to an inquiry or investigation by a state licensing board; (c) court orders, such as when a psychological or custody evaluation is court ordered, notwithstanding the legal precedent that the confidential communications during psychotherapy sessions are otherwise privileged under federal and state law; (d) serious, imminent, and foreseeable danger of violence to the client or others; and (e) worker's compensation cases, when authorized by the client and to the extent necessary to comply with laws relating to worker's compensation or other similar programs.

Perhaps one of the most comprehensive approaches to informed consent has been outlined by Schlosser and Tower (1991), who require their clients to read and initial each page of a 10-page description of office policies and procedures. Schlosser and Tower observe, "Prior to using written policies, we would on occasion encounter a difference of opinion regarding expectations, cost, billing procedures, and third-party coverage. Adoption of these materials has reduced such problems significantly" (p. 393).

For counselors, an excellent template is contained in G. Corey and colleagues' (2007, pp. 182-187) six-page Sample Informed Consent Document, which contains a particularly detailed description of informed consent procedures relevant to working with children and adolescents. Although the sample form is very lengthy, it provides valuable information that can be used by counselors developing their own informed consent documents.

For psychologists, an excellent resource that has become the industry standard is the APAIT Psychotherapist-Patient Contract promoted by Eric Harris and Bruce Bennett (Bennett et al., 1997; Harris, 2004). The seven-page Psychotherapist-Patient Contract covers information such as the scope of psychological services, length of meetings, professional fees, billing and payments, insurance reimbursement, therapist contact information, record storage and retention, patient access to records, exceptions to confidentiality, and special consideration of issues related to the treatment of minors. The APAIT contract is recommended as a way to reduce liability risk by managing client expectations from the outset. The contract is available at http://www.apait.org.*

Regarding financial arrangements, APA Ethical Standard 6.04(a) (Fees and Financial Arrangements) states, "As early as is feasible in a professional or scientific relationship, psychologists and recipients of psychological services reach an agreement specifying compensation and billing arrangements" (2002, p. 1068). Such an agreement might include a discussion of fees, payment for missed sessions, billing for phone calls and letters, the use of collection agencies, and financial arrangements should the client lose his or her source of income (Handelsman & Galvin, 1988). In the practice of managed care, an informed consent discussion might also include contractual agreements, precertification requirements, limitations in coverage, and termination procedures (G. Corey et al., 2007; Younggren, 1995). Clinicians should provide enough information for the client to make informed decisions, but not so much information that the client becomes confused and overwhelmed. As a practical guideline regarding how much significant information to discuss, Haas and Malouf (2005) advise, "If in doubt, inform the person anyway. It is always better to [have provided sufficient information] than to be accused later of having denied the patient the opportunity to decide for himself or herself" (p. 67). Again, remember the Golden Rule of informed consent by considering how much information you would want provided to you if you were in the client's seat.

AVOID UNDUE INFLUENCE

The third element of informed consent requires that the client's consent must be obtained freely and without "undue influence." The psychologist must determine whether the client has provided consent on an adequately voluntary basis. This would mean that there has been no coercion or undue influence based on the client's vulnerable condition or other factors (Canter et al., 1994).

Some legal analysts have pointed out that competent and adequately informed consent "will be presumed to be freely given unless there is a *specific indication of fraud, coercion or duress*" (Stromberg et al., 1988, p. 450). Nevertheless, psychologists should remain alert to subtle ways

---

* Although all websites cited in this book were correct at the time of publication, they are subject to change at any time.

in which undue influence may unwittingly occur, such as emphasizing the benefits while failing to mention the risks of psychotherapy. At the same time, psychologists must decide how "risky" a psychotherapeutic procedure might be before informing a client of the risk in the first place. When discussing such risks with their clients, psychologists must be reasonable and sensitive in presenting the information in a way that does not unduly influence the client's decision (Andrews, 1984). In some cases, it may be advisable to discuss the *limitations* rather than the risks of therapy. Stromberg et al. (1988) advise psychologists to inform their therapy clients of "the type of therapy, the approximate length of time the treatment may require, the cost of treatment, and any substantial risks or side effects that might reasonably occur as a result of the treatment" (p. 449). Because treatment is an ongoing process, the client must also adequately understand and voluntarily agree to any changes in the ongoing treatment plan.

OBTAIN WRITTEN
DOCUMENTATION

The fourth and final element of the informed consent process requires the clinician "appropriately document" the client's consent. It is important to point out that APA Ethical Standards do *not* require a signed consent form. However, Ethical Standard 3.10(d) (Informed Consent) does require that "Psychologists appropriately document written or oral consent, permission, and assent" (p. 1065). Whether one chooses a more casual question-answer format or a formal, written narrative approach, compliance with APA standards requires that the client's consent be appropriately documented. Appropriate documentation can range from a signed informed consent form to a brief progress note that records the basic matters discussed (Canter et al., 1994). Most ethicists recommend the use of a detailed, signed informed consent form (Bennett et al., 1995, 1996, 2006; Piazza & Yeager, 1991; Shapiro, 1994; Younggren, 1995, 2006). Piazza and Baruth (1990) point out that a signed authorization provides clear evidence that the psychologist and the client "have discussed the treatment to be provided, its potential benefits, potential limitations, and a statement that the client has given his or her consent to be treated" (p. 315). A flexible approach combining both verbal discussion and written documentation may offer more protection than either method alone.

Consistent with Handelsman and Galvin's (1988) question-discussion format, Stromberg et al. (1988) suggest that the psychologist present to the client a general informed consent form that discloses basic information, with space provided for the psychologist to write in detail or in summary what else was discussed. The form can be signed and initialed by the client. For example, the Sample Informed Consent Form illustrated in G. Corey et al. (2007) contains places where the client can initial various sections of the form before signing the complete document. The combined verbal discussion and written documentation approach "provides persuasive evidence that a conscientious effort to obtain informed consent was made" (Stromberg et al., 1988, p. 451). Stromberg et al. (1988) also describe another option: a two-step process in which a consent form is supplemented by oral discussion, leading to a written statement by the client designed to demonstrate the client's understanding of the information. The "written statement" approach has been described as particularly useful because courts have focused most closely on the client's understanding, even though it constitutes only one component of competency.

The consent forms contained on the CD-ROM accompanying this book represent a formal method for appropriately documenting discussion of the basic elements of informed consent. Other appropriate forms are available in resources such as *The Paper Office* (Zuckerman, 2002) and *The Clinical Documentation Sourcebook: The Complete Paperwork Resource for Your Mental Health Practice* (Wiger, 2005).

NOTE EXCEPTIONS TO INFORMED CONSENT

There are four exceptions to the requirement to obtain informed consent, which are described in *The Psychologist's Legal Handbook* (Stromberg et al., 1988). One exception includes situations in which the client expressly and specifically waives the right. Such a waiver should be "knowing" or informed. In order to ensure that the waiver is "knowing" or informed, Stromberg and associates explain that patients should be told that the psychologist "is willing to inform the patient about the treatment, unless the patient would rather that the therapist not inform him, and this should be carefully documented" (p. 452). Stromberg and Dellinger (1993) discuss three other situations in which "informed consent may be reduced or dispensed: (1) in emergencies, either affecting the individual's or the public's health or safety; (2) when the patient lacks the ability to understand or agree, in which case someone else must consent for him; and (3) when disclosure would harm the patient" (pp. 6-7). This last exception, which is also known as "therapeutic privilege," applies when the psychologist intentionally does not inform a patient of certain facts because to do so would harm the patient. Legal precedent for invoking "therapeutic privilege" is based on court decisions that have found that information can be withheld from a patient "when the disclosure poses such a threat of detriment to the patient as to become infeasible or contra-indicated from a medical point of view" (*Canterbury v. Spence,* 1972). However, Stromberg and Dellinger (1993) have noted that most legal writers have cautioned against invoking therapeutic privilege except in "extraordinarily justifiable situations" (p. 6).

An exception to the doctrine of informed consent exists in emergency situations in which there may be a danger to the health or safety of the patient or others. In cases involving emergency situations, "Psychologists should attempt to obtain the best possible version of informed consent in all cases, even when treating distressed patients" (Stromberg et al., 1988, p. 452). One recommendation would be to discuss with each new patient basic reasons for seeking treatment, anticipated costs, treatment effects, and confidentiality issues "*as soon as clinically advisable*" (Stromberg et al., 1988, p. 451). Although APA Ethical Principles do not directly address exceptions to informed consent in emergency situations, psychologists are advised to consult with colleagues when dispensing with informed consent in certain research situations. Consultation with a colleague is advisable in situations in which the client is unable to give consent (Canter et al., 1994). In medical emergencies, it may also be advisable for the psychologist to obtain input from significant others. Procedural guidelines might include consideration of the patient's best interests, consultation with a peer, obtaining information from next of kin or significant others, and discussion with the client as soon as it is clinically advisable. In any event, dispensing with informed consent should be considered the exception rather than the rule.

As discussed earlier, there is an exception to the requirement for obtaining informed consent from legally "incompetent" clients, including minor children. Informed consent procedures for such individuals are addressed by APA Ethical Standards that allow "substitute consent" as permitted by law. Substitute consent allows the psychologist to obtain consent from a legally authorized person, such as the parent of a minor child or the guardian of an incompetent person. Even in such situations, however, the child and particularly the mature minor or older adolescent client have certain rights to know what is happening. The psychologist has an ethical duty to explain the procedures, seek the child's assent, and consider the child's preferences and best interests.

Therapists working with children must maintain a delicate balance between protecting the child's ethical rights to privacy, required to build trust necessary to create a therapeutic relationship with the child, and honoring the parents' legal rights to information about their child's treatment. As G. Corey et al. (2007) point out, although child clients have ethical rights to privacy and confidentiality in the counseling relationship, in most cases laws favor the legal rights of parents over their children. Although parental rights may vary according to specific state statutes (Remley & Herlihy, 2005), it is important to manage expectations from the outset by reaching a mutually acceptable agreement regarding the exceptions to confidentiality and the extent that confidential information will be shared with the parents of a minor child involved in therapy. As G. Corey et al. (2007) caution, "If the matter of confidentiality is not clearly explored with all parties involved, it is almost certain that problems will emerge in the course of therapy" (p. 191). Lawrence and Robinson-Kurpius (2000) recommend that counselors involve the parents in the initial meeting with their child in order to arrive at a mutual agreement regarding the nature and extent of information that will be provided to them by the therapist during the course of counseling of their child.

In the case of mature minors, there are generally three ways that therapists handle information disclosed by older adolescent clients, including (a) *complete confidentiality*, in which the therapist maintains complete confidentiality and does not disclose any information to the parents; (b) *no confidentiality*, in which the therapist discloses all information given to the therapist by the adolescent; and (c) *limited confidentiality*, in which the therapist uses professional judgment and reserves the right to disclose information to the parents based on the best interests of the child. The limited confidentiality policy offers the most flexibility and allows the greatest latitude in professional judgment than either of the two more extreme positions. In general, most therapists refuse to keep certain information secret (e.g., behavior that is dangerous or destructive toward the client or others) because such secrets can otherwise contribute to triangulation and create ethical dilemmas for the therapist. Lawrence and Robinson-Kurpius (2000) use the term *informed forced consent* to refer to another option for handling information during sessions with minor children. In informed forced consent, the therapist does not make any guarantee of confidentiality to the adolescent client, the adolescent has no say in what is disclosed to parents, but the adolescent is given advance notice before any disclosure is made to the parents. Of course, this option makes it even more important for the therapist to have obtained the adolescent's advance understanding and agreement before this type of policy can be used, although this option does not truly involve consent because consent is not voluntarily given by the adolescent. Regardless of which of the preceding policies the therapist prefers, the most important ethical considerations involve creating realistic client expectations in advance through the initial informed consent discussion with all parties (adolescent and parents) and through the ongoing process of communication with the client.

CONSIDER
LEGAL STANDARDS

Although questions have been raised about whether informed consent procedures provide any protection against legal liability, there is no question that *failure* to obtain informed consent is a proven area of legal risk (Stromberg & Dellinger, 1993). Court rulings have shown that practitioners who fail to obtain informed consent may be held liable for a breach of the standard of care (e.g., *Canterbury v. Spence,* 1972; *Clites v. Iowa,* 1980). Stromberg and Dellinger (1993) have pointed out, "Because the patient's informed consent is deemed to have a value in itself, psychologists can be held liable for failure to obtain appropriate informed consent *even if their subsequent treatment of the patient is exemplary from a clinical perspective*" (p. 5). In an age of litigation, psychologists are advised to obtain informed consent that is detailed, discussed, and signed (Bennett et al., 1995, 1996; Piazza & Baruth, 1990; Younggren, 1995, 2006). Because such documentation provides a record for the future, most legal analysts recommend the use of a written consent form (Stromberg et al., 1988). Piazza and Baruth (1990) recommend that such authorization be obtained "from every client before or at the time of the first visit" (p. 315). On the other hand, Schlosser and Tower (1991) recommend that their clients take home and review their 10-page office policy form, emphasizing, "Handing out these lengthy materials before a first meeting with a client would likely appear too bureaucratic and impersonal" (p. 393). In using the APAIT Psychotherapist-Patient Contract, many therapists provide a brief discussion of the document and have the client take the form home and read it before returning, discussing, and signing the document in the presence of the therapist during the next session (Younggren, 2006).

As Piazza and Yeager (1991) have observed, "Psychotherapy is increasingly being viewed as a hazardous or invasive procedure, and having a signed statement of informed consent can help reduce the risk of litigation following a negative treatment experience" (p. 344). The use of a written consent form is especially important "if consent is given on behalf of another (such as a minor child) or is a consent for innovative, confrontational, or risky therapies" (Stromberg et al., 1988, p. 447). On a related matter, it is interesting to note that at one time the APAIT professional liability insurance policy required that psychologists who offered services "involving physical contact" with clients to submit a copy of their "release form" with their insurance renewal application (APAIT, 1996, p. 2). As a general rule, the more invasive or innovative the procedure, the greater the need for adequately informed consent and careful documentation of procedures.

CONSIDER
FEDERAL REGULATIONS

An important set of legal standards has also been brought about by the Health Insurance Portability and Accountability Act (HIPAA), which came into being as a result of passage of the Kassenbaum-Kennedy bill that was signed into law as PL104-191 in 1996. Designed to help contain the ever-rising health care costs by streamlining the system through the adoption of standards for transmitting electronic health care claims, HIPAA regulations also establish standards for protecting the privacy of medical records. The national standards imposed by HIPAA affect all health service providers. Whether mental health professionals like it or not, HIPAA federal regulations are so broad and comprehensive that they have become the new national standard of care for privacy, record retention, and authorizations for disclosure. Although an analysis of HIPAA is beyond the scope of this book, HIPAA compliant practitioners must have formal policies, procedures, and practices designed to protect the privacy of health information. At a bare minimum, the Privacy Rule requires that such policies must address the uses and disclosures of protected health information (PHI) for treatment, payment, and health care operations; a description of the uses and disclosures requiring patient authorization; a description of the uses and disclosures requiring neither consent nor authorization; and a description of the patient's rights and the practitioner's duties. The Security Rule and the Transaction Rule impose more complex requirements, which are beyond the scope of this book.

As Zur (2003) has pointed out, HIPAA is the standard of care by which all mental health professionals will be judged regardless of their billing practices or their technical status as "covered entities." Zur has identified three types of clinicians with respect to HIPAA: possums, ostriches, and eagles. Overwhelmed by the demands of HIPAA, some clinicians respond by rolling over and playing dead like possums, whereas others respond by hiding their heads in the sand like ostriches. The appropriate response to HIPAA is to be an alert and vigilant eagle. Despite the April 14, 2003 deadline of the Privacy Rule and the Security Rule, as well as the October 15, 2003 deadline of the Transaction Rule, many clinicians in private practice settings are still not HIPAA compliant. As Zuckerman has pointed out, "Courts may view the Privacy Rule as setting the standard for protecting PHI and so, in a lawsuit or state licensing board complaint, the practitioner will be judged by HIPAA's rules as the standards" (2003, p. 17). Like it or not, HIPAA is the standard of care for health care providers.

CONSIDER
MANAGED CARE

The practice of managed care raises some complex informed consent issues. Several of these issues are summarized by Younggren (1995), who notes that insured clients who actually understand their benefits packages are usually the exception rather than the rule. To complicate matters further, Acuff et al. (1999) point out that some managed care organizations make it a practice not to provide full, complete, and accurate disclosures of information to their insureds. The implication is that many clients have no idea of how their policies affect their patient rights, access to insurance benefits, and amount of service received under these plans. Clients who think they have unlimited insurance benefits are typically unaware that their maximum benefits are rarely authorized by their managed care company reviewers. For this reason, when discussing financial arrangements with the client, it may be helpful to explain differences between health insurance and managed care so that the client can better appreciate how his or her particular plan operates (Doverspike, 1995). Although insurance verification and managed care precertification have become standard operating procedures for most mental health providers during the past decade, many clients do not understand that their therapists may have to obtain prior authorization for psychotherapy and related procedures (Younggren, 1995, 2006). It is a mistake to assume that new clients have been given complete information by their insurance companies regarding how a managed care policy will affect the services they receive (Acuff et al., 1999).

In cases involving diagnostic assessment, procedures such as psychological testing typically require prior authorization and sometimes require submission of the written report to the managed care company.

Most clients are surprised to learn that their managed care company will have access to confidential information such as outpatient treatment reports (OTR), telephone reviews, email communications, and occasionally even progress notes. There are occasions when it may be advisable to have the client present during telephone precertification or utilization reviews (Doverspike, 1995). Having the client present during such calls can improve communication, encourage a collaborative atmosphere, and provide the client with a better understanding of the review process.

Given the managed care treatment philosophy of short-term crisis intervention, psychologists are obliged to discuss at the outset of therapy issues related to termination and limitations of services (Younggren, 1995). Regarding limitations to services that can be anticipated because of limitations in financing, APA (2002) Ethical Standard 10.01(a) (Informed Consent to Therapy) requires that this be discussed with the client or other appropriate recipient of services "as early as is feasible" (p. 1072). Regarding interruption of services, APA (2002) Ethical Standard 10.09 (Interruption of Therapy) requires that psychologists provide for appropriate resolution of responsibility of client care "in the event that the employment or contractual relationship ends, with paramount consideration given to the welfare of the client/patient" (p. 1073). Given the preference of many managed care clients to continue receiving services beyond those authorized as "clinically necessary" by their case managers, it is important to manage the client's expectations from the outset. When structuring the therapy relationship and anticipating a limit in the number of sessions authorized or financed by a managed care company, the prudent practitioner discusses options in advance. These options may include consideration of time-limited sessions, termination when initial goals are achieved, referral to a public mental health center, as well as the option of client self-payment. Most managed care contracts permit the client to self-pay for services that are not considered clinically necessary *if* such an arrangement is clarified and agreed upon in advance. The CD-ROM accompanying this book contains various consent forms that can be used to document the client's understanding of professional services that may be provided in the absence of clinical necessity.

USE INFORMED
CONSENT FORMS

Because informed consent is an ongoing, dynamic, and continuing process of informing the client about what may be required, the written consent forms should never be a substitute for ongoing discussion with the client. Merely having a client "sign off" on several forms at intake is not sufficient to have properly established informed consent. Written consent forms should always be accompanied by a discussion of the issues to ensure the client's understanding (G. Corey et al., 2007; Handelsman & Galvin, 1988; Schlosser & Tower, 1991; Younggren, 2005, 2006).

With regard to the development of an appropriate consent form, it should be emphasized that the consent forms contained on the CD-ROM accompanying this book do not represent static documents, but, rather, each form represents one frame in an ongoing process of development. Beginning with a prototype consent form developed several years ago, the consent forms have undergone literally dozens of revisions based on legal advice, peer consultation, revised ethical principles, and evolving standards of practice. Each paragraph reflects a situation and each sentence addresses a question that has arisen in my own clinical practice. A useful consent form strikes a balance between general and specific information. As Handelsman and Galvin (1988) observe, "It is hard to avoid some information that is so specific that it does not apply to many clients or so general that it conveys almost nothing" (p. 224).

Some of the consent forms contained on the CD-ROM were originally designed for my hospital practice that includes diagnostic consultations, psychological assessment, neuropsychological testing, and brief psychotherapy. Because diagnostic and assessment services are often requested by a third party such as a referring physician, some of the consent forms contained on the CD-ROM place an emphasis on standards related to limits of confidentiality and release of information. The reader is encouraged to modify these forms and develop templates that are more appropriate for use in his or her practice. Several of the consent forms also address other areas of practice. Documentation of informed consent for evaluations is particularly important in the case of forensic testimony, child custody evaluations, and independent consultative examinations, because such evaluations are often associated with litigation and professional liability complaints.

Although these forms specify "psychologist" as the provider, the forms can be easily modified for other mental health professionals. Depending on the provider's preferences, terms such as "patient" may also be substituted for "client," and the descriptions of services may be modified to fit one's practice. These forms provide basic significant information that can be discussed with the client to ensure the client's understanding. In cases where certain information should be emphasized to the client, the psychologist may choose to underline the material and have the client place his or her initials next to such sections. In cases where the client may object to certain conditions, the psychologist has the option of striking through a section that can be initialed by the provider and client. In cases where the client raises several objections or refuses to sign the form, the psychologist should consider the implications of the client's actions in deciding whether to provide services under such circumstances.

Because these forms were designed specifically for an assessment-oriented practice, the forms do not address all of the issues that may arise as part of an ongoing informed consent discussion in other types of practices. The forms can be modified and customized as needed for other specialty practices and procedures. Some practitioners may prefer the use of a generic form that can be tailored for each client by filling in specific information, while others may prefer to use a series of separate paragraphs, forms, or brochures that address relevant issues as they arise. Other areas of informed consent discussion include basic issues such as cancelation policies, emergency and weekend coverage, the use of telephone consultations, and online counseling.

In the practice of managed care, issues related to the release of specific information may require ongoing discussion and documentation of informed consent. In the case of Outpatient Treatment Reports (OTR), it is usually helpful to have the patient sign the bottom of the OTR after he or she has reviewed and approved the information to be released to the managed care company. More detailed informed consent procedures might be required for more complex clinical situations such as child custody evaluations, independent consultative examinations, biofeedback treatment, or the use of hypnosis or other specialized procedures. Therapists working in more controversial areas such as "recovered memories" would be well advised to consult with their attorneys regarding appropriate informed consent procedures.

Sample consent forms are contained on the CD-ROM accompanying this book. These consent forms and the contents of the CD-ROM and this book are not intended to provide legal advice and the information contained in them should not be relied upon for legal advice. The reader is encouraged to contact a qualified attorney for legal advice regarding state and federal laws governing informed consent.

SUMMARY OF INFORMED CONSENT CONSIDERATIONS

To use an old proverb, "An ounce of prevention is worth a pound of cure." From a risk-management perspective, informed consent procedures help prevent ethical problems before they arise. Written consent forms provide a means of documenting informed consent, but such forms should never be used as a substitute for sound legal advice and a working knowledge of ethical principles. When used appropriately, written consent forms can provide some helpful guidelines for facilitating open communication, ongoing discussion, clarification of choices, and decision making.

POINTS TO REMEMBER

- Determine the client's capacity to give consent.
- Assume the client is competent unless there is evidence to the contrary.
- Provide enough significant information for the client to make a decision.
- Manage client expectations from the outset of therapy.
- Avoid undue influence in the client's decision-making process.
- Obtain written documentation of informed decisions.
- Consider the use of formal informed consent documents.

Chapter Three

Managing Boundaries: Staying Off the Slippery Slope

Whenever I think of boundaries, I think of the "shoebox case." The case involved a former psychotherapy patient who filed a written complaint that was accompanied by a shoebox filled with cards, love letters, photographs, and other evidence to support the patient's complaint of having had a sexualized dual relationship with the psychotherapist. The investigation of the complaint revealed that the alleged sexual relationship had been the culmination of a long history of multiple boundary violations. Yet when the boundary violations were traced back to their origin, the first step down the slippery slope seemed to be a subtle boundary crossing that itself was not unethical. The case was my first glimpse into the inner world of a psychotherapist who was living a nightmare of a downward spiral that had begun with a simple step across a boundary.

If good fences make good neighbors, as the proverb goes, then good boundaries make a firm foundation for a good relationship in psychotherapy. A boundary is the edge or limit of appropriate behavior in a given situation. What is the difference between a boundary crossing and a boundary violation? A *boundary crossing* is a change in role or a departure from a commonly accepted practice that could potentially benefit a client, whereas a *boundary violation* is an ethical breach that harms or exploits the client at some level (Gutheil & Gabbard, 1993). Lazarus and Zur (2002) describe a boundary crossing as a "benign and often beneficial departure from traditional therapeutic settings or constraints" (p. 6), whereas a boundary violation involves therapist actions "that are harmful, exploitative, or in direct conflict with the preservation of clients' dignity and the integrity of the therapeutic process" (p. 6).

45

Boundary crossings are not necessarily unethical, but boundary violations are *always* unethical. An example of a boundary crossing would be giving your last client of the day a ride to the bus stop when it is pouring down rain, in order to provide some benefit to the client. The therapist's behavior in this example is not a form of exploitation because the behavior is primarily designed to benefit the client—not the therapist. Of course, the problem with a boundary crossing is that it could lead to loss of effectiveness with the client or loss of objectivity on the part of the therapist. Although boundary crossings are not necessarily unethical, another problem with boundary crossings is that they may lead to boundary violations. An example of a boundary violation would be asking your last client of the day for a ride to the bus stop when it is pouring down rain, in order to provide some benefit to you. The therapist's request in this example is a form of exploitation because the request is primarily designed to benefit the therapist—not the client. If there is any benefit to the client, it is incidental (rather than intentional) to the boundary violation. From an ethical risk-management perspective, the best way to avoid boundary violations is to avoid boundary crossings. Boundary crossings can occur in several ways, including dual relationships, incidental encounters, role-blending, stealth dilemmas, ethical blind spots, and hybrid relationships. The conscientious practitioner is able to identify boundary crossings and manage boundaries appropriately from the outset.

DUAL RELATIONSHIPS

Ethical problems often arise when therapists blend their professional relationship with other kinds of relationships. Dual or multiple role relationships occur when a professional assumes two or more roles at the same time or sequentially with a client or with someone who has a significant relationship with the client. I prefer the use of the term *dual relationships* rather than the politically correct but the less accurate term *multiple relationships*. In reality, most boundary crossings involve a duality, rather than a multiplicity, of roles. Even when multiple roles are involved, there is always a dual role before there are multiple roles. In other words, there must be two roles before there can be three or more. There must be a primary role before there can be a secondary role, and there must be a secondary role before there can be a tertiary role, and so on. From the perspective of aspirational ethics, the clinician striving for excellence in boundary management pays attention to maintaining the integrity of boundaries in the primary professional role. If the primary role is managed appropriately, then secondary roles are less likely to develop in the first place. If secondary roles do develop, they are less likely to become problematic.

Dual Roles Defined

APA (2002, p. 1065) Ethical Standard 3.05 (Multiple Relationships) states the following:

(a) A multiple relationship occurs when a psychologist is in a professional role with a person and (1) at the same time is in another role with the same person, (2) at the same time is in a relationship with a person closely associated with or related to the person with whom the psychologist has the professional relationship, or (3) promises to enter into another relationship in the future with the person or a person closely associated with or related to the person.

A psychologist refrains from entering into a multiple relationship if the multiple relationship could reasonably be expected to impair the psychologist's objectivity, com-petence, or effectiveness in performing his or her functions as a psychologist, or otherwise risks exploitation or harm to the person with whom the professional relationship exists.

Multiple relationships that would not reasonably be expected to cause impairment or risk exploitation or harm are not unethical.

(b) If a psychologist finds that, due to unforeseen factors, a potentially harmful multiple relationship has arisen, the psychologist takes reasonable steps to resolve it with due regard for the best interests of the affected person and maximal compliance with the Ethics Code.

(c) When psychologists are required by law, institutional policy, or extraordinary circumstances to serve in more than one role in judicial or administrative proceedings, at the outset they clarify role expectations and the extent of confidentiality and thereafter as changes occur. (See also Standards 3.04, Avoiding Harm, and 3.07, Third-Party Requests for Services.)

Foreseeable and
Unforeseeable Dual Roles

Dual roles differ in terms of their predictability or foreseeability. Dual roles can be classified as either foreseeable or unforeseeable. *Foreseeable* (or contemplated) dual roles are those that the therapist has time to consider or contemplate before engaging in them. An example of a foreseeable dual role would involve considering whether or not to provide psychotherapy to someone with whom you have had a prior social or business relationship (such as one of the fitness trainers or members at your gym). *Unforeseeable* (unpredictable, or random) dual roles are those that cannot be reasonably foreseen. Using the above examples, an unforeseeable role might involve joining a gym and later learning that one of the fitness instructors or gym members is one of your former clients. Of course, if you had prior knowledge that your psychotherapy client was also a fitness instructor or gym member, then the subsequent dual role may have been reasonably foreseeable. This framework of classifying dual roles along the dimension of foreseeability is not meant to imply that any of the preceding roles are ethical or unethical, but simply to clarify the different ways in which dual roles can develop.

In the case of foreseeable or contemplated dual relationships, APA (2002) Ethical Standard 3.05(a) contains a caution: "A psychologist refrains from entering into a multiple relationship if the multiple relationship *could reasonably be expected* [italics added] to impair the psychologist's objectivity, competence, or effectiveness in performing his or her functions as a psychologist, or otherwise risks exploitation or harm to the person with whom the professional relationship exists" (p. 1065). In those dual relationships in which a client eventually perceives harm or exploitation, the burden of proof will fall on the psychologist to demonstrate that the prospective relationship could not reasonably have been expected to result in harm. Adjudication of licensing board complaints is often determined partly by the way that disciplinary boards interpret the meaning of the phrase "could reasonably be expected." The word "reasonably" does not define itself. What is reasonable to one psychologist may not be reasonable to another. These considerations highlight the importance of consulting with colleagues in situations involving dual roles or boundary crossings. Of course, the best way to stay out of deep water is to avoid the slippery slope in the first place.

G. Corey et al. (2007, p. 275) suggest that counselors ask the simple question, "In what way is what I am contemplating in the best interest of the client?" Lazarus and Zur (2002) provide dozens of practical guidelines related to dual relationships, the first of which states, "Always do whatever it takes to help clients" (p. 473). With respect to contemplated dual relationships, Gottlieb (1993) advises that the therapists consider three dimensions of the current professional relationship: (a) power differential, (b) duration of relationship, and (c) specificity of termination. The first step involves assessing the current relationship according to the three dimensions of power differential (low, mid-range, and high power), duration of relationship (brief, intermediate, long duration), and specificity of termination (specific, uncertain, and indefinite termination). From the perspective of the client, where does the relationship fall on each of these dimensions? The second step involves examining the contemplated relationship along the three dimensions, as was done for the current relationship. The third step involves examining both relationships for role incompatibility if they fall within the mid-range or to the left side (e.g., low power differential, brief duration, and specific termination) of the dimensions. The final step involves obtaining consultation from a colleague before proceeding with the contemplated secondary relationship.

In the case of unforeseeable dual relationships, APA (2002) Ethical Standard 3.05(b) states, "If a psychologist finds that, due to unforeseen factors, a potentially harmful multiple relationship has arisen, the psychologist takes reasonable steps to resolve it with due regard for the best interests of the affected person and maximal compliance with the Ethics Code" (p. 1065). Resolving the dilemma of duality may include several options such as discussing the matter with the client, consulting with a colleague, considering termination of the secondary role, considering termination of the primary professional role, and so forth. Regardless of the option, the ultimate ethics question is, "What is in the best interest of the client?"

Concurrent and Consecutive Dual Roles

Dual roles can also be classified as either concurrent or consecutive in time. *Concurrent* (or simultaneous) dual roles exist when a therapist has two roles at the same time with the same client, or with a person who is in a significant relationship with the client. In other words, the two roles occur simultaneously. For example, a concurrent or simultaneous dual role might involve beginning family therapy and then later learning that one of the members of the family is currently on your child's soccer team. *Consecutive* (or sequential) dual roles involve a prior relationship that involves either a professional or nonprofessional role followed by the development of a second relationship at a later point in time. An example of a consecutive or sequential dual role might involve joining a gym and later learning that one of the fitness instructors is one of your former clients, in which the professional relationship was primary and then the business or social role developed secondarily. Another example might involve a situation in which the social or business role came first, such as providing psychotherapy to someone with whom you have had a prior social or business relationship (such as one of the fitness trainers at the gym). This classification of dual roles along the dimension of time is not meant to suggest that any of the above roles are ethical or unethical, but simply to illustrate the different ways in which dual roles can develop.

Table 1: Types of Dual Relationships

	Foreseeable	**Unforeseeable**
Concurrent	Foreseeable Concurrent	Unforeseeable Concurrent
Consecutive	Foreseeable Consecutive	Unforeseeable Consecutive

Table 1 (above) depicts four types of dual relationships, each of which is illustrated by one of the following examples: A *foreseeable concurrent* dual role might involve considering whether to provide therapy to your personal trainer or a member of the gym where you take an exercise class, whereas an *unforeseeable concurrent* dual relationship might involve learning that one of your psychotherapy clients is married to your personal trainer or a member of the gym where you take an exercise class. A *foreseeable consecutive* dual relationship might involve considering whether to provide psychotherapy to your former personal trainer or a former member of the gym where you take an exercise class, whereas an *unforeseeable consecutive* dual relationship might involve learning that your personal trainer or member of your gym is one of your former psychotherapy clients. Again, this framework of classifying dual relationships is not meant to imply that any of the previous types of relationships is ethical or unethical, but simply to clarify the different ways in which dual roles can develop.

Normalization of
Dual Roles

In the last decade, there has been a trend toward neutralization of the implied ethicality of some types of dual relationships. This trend is particularly noticeable in the comparisons between the 1992 and 2002 versions of the APA *Ethical Principles of Psychologists and Code of Conduct* as well as between the 1995 and 2005 versions of the ACA *Code of Ethics*. For example, the wording of the 1992 APA Ethics Code implied that multiple relationships were inherently unethical, which essentially placed the burden of proof on any psychologist who was charged with having engaged in a dual relationship—unethical or otherwise. In contrast, the 2002 APA Ethical Standard 3.05 (Multiple Relationships) simply begins with a neutral definition of a multiple relationship. After providing a neutral definition of a multiple relation-ship, Ethical Standard 3.05(a) unequivocally states, "Multiple relation-ships that would not reasonably be expected to cause impairment or risk exploitation or harm are not unethical" (p. 1065).

There has been a trend toward liberalization of boundaries seen in the publication of books such as Lazarus and Zur's (2002) *Dual Relationships and Psychotherapy*, which at first glance perhaps should have been titled *Boundary Violations and Psychotherapy*. As one reviewer has noted, "At first glance, it is a book of ethical heresy that challenges the uncontested dogma of ethical conservatism" (Doverspike, 2004a, p. 209). Lazarus and Zur's book abounds with examples of nonsexual boundary crossings, role-blending, and so-called "hybrid relationships." Lazarus and Zur (2002) make the point that duality in relationships should not be confused with exploitation. Just as an ethical therapist can engage in some nonsexual dual roles without risking exploitation or harm to the client, an unethical therapist can exploit or harm a client without engaging in any type of dual role at all. Notwithstanding the unconventional perspectives of some of the authors who contributed to *Dual Relationships and Psychotherapy,* the publication of such a book itself represents an example of the increasing liberalization of the concept of dual relationships.

Although it is clear that Lazarus and Zur do not advocate boundary violations, they do advocate boundary crossings that may sometimes benefit clients. Lest one reject their position without careful consideration of their arguments, it may be helpful to identify the common ground that Lazarus and Zur share with even the most conservative ethicists. First, in the Introduction section of *Dual Relationships and Psychotherapy*, Lazarus and Zur clearly support the majority opinion that "Sexual activities are obviously and appropriately forbidden" (p. xxvii). The universal prohibition against sexual relations with clients is a theme that is repeated throughout their book. Lazarus and Zur also state that dual relationships are unethical if they involve conflicts of interest, such as a teacher serving as a therapist to students graded by the teacher. The authors also maintain a position that is "totally opposed to any form of disparagement, exploitation, abuse, or harassment" (p. 29). Finally, Lazarus and Zur note that "it is inadvisable to disregard strict boundary limits" in the presence of severe psychopathology, involving "passive-aggressive, histrionic, or manipulative behaviors; borderline personality features; or manifestations of suspiciousness and undue hostility" (p. 27). At least in these respects, the underlying ethical foundation of *Dual Relationships and Psychotherapy* is within the mainstream of even the most conservative ethicists.

Partly as a result of the liberalization of dual roles in the APA Code of Conduct, there has been a trend toward liberalization of state licensing board rules governing boundaries. For example, in neutralizing the definition of dual relationships, the 2004 revision of the Georgia Rules eliminated the so-called "hammer clause" that had previously been contained in Chapter 510-5-.05 (1), titled as "Dual Relationship Affecting Psychologist's Judgment," of the 1996 Rules of the State Board of Examiners of Psychologists:

> The psychologist shall not undertake or continue a professional relationship with a client, supervisee, employee, research participant, or student when the objectivity or competency of the psychologist is, or could reasonably be expected by the Board to be, impaired because of the psychologist's present or previous familial, social, emotional, supervisory, political, administrative, or legal relationship with the client, or a relevant person associated with or related to the client. If such dual relationship develops or is discovered after the professional relationship has been initiated, the psychologist is in violation of the Code of Conduct and shall terminate the professional relationship in an appropriate manner, shall notify the client in writing of this termination, shall assist

the client in obtaining services from another professional, and shall not engage in any self-enhancing relationship with the client until at least a period of 24 months has elapsed after the termination. (Rules of the State Board of Examiners of Psychologists, Chapter 510-5.05 [1], 1996).*

Review of Literature

Although authors of ethics articles in APA journals generally use the term *multiple relationships*, writers in ACA literature typically use the terms *dual roles* and *role-blending*. One of the most cited articles on this subject in the field of counseling is St. Germaine's (1993) "Dual relationships: What's wrong with them?" Perhaps the best review of the literature on role-blending and dual relationships in the field of counseling is provided by Herlihy and G. Corey's (1997) book, *Boundary Issues in Counseling: Multiple Roles and Responsibilities.* Herlihy and G. Corey identify 10 key themes surrounding multiple roles in counseling relationships. A summary of these reviews is contained in G. Corey et al.'s (2007) textbook *Issues and Ethics in the Helping Professions*, which itself is arguably one of the most widely used ethics textbooks in the field of counseling.

In the field of psychology, perhaps the most comprehensive resource would be Koocher and Keith-Spiegel's (1998) textbook *Ethics in Psychology: Professional Standards and Cases.* Koocher and Keith-Spiegel provide an excellent blend of academic scholarship and common sense in what has been described as the first comprehensive reference book on ethics in psychology. Another choice is Haas and Malouf's (2005) textbook, *Keeping Up the Good Work: A Practitioner's Guide to Mental Health Ethics,* which contains sporadic scholarly citations but a multitude of practical guidelines and questions for practitioners to ask themselves when working in actual clinical practice. Designed less as a textbook and more as the practical handbook suggested by its subtitle, Haas and Malouf's book contains a chapter devoted to the topics of dual relationships, avoiding exploitation, and maintaining appropriate

---

* The 1996 revision of the Georgia Rules of the State Board of Examiners of Psychologists refers to the Rules that were revised on April 18, 1996. These Rules were previously adopted and filed on July 27, 1994 and became effective August 16, 1994. Following the publication of the APA (2002) *Ethical Principles of Psychologists and Code of Conduct*, the Georgia State Board of Examiners of Psychologists adopted the APA Code of Ethics and also added a Supplemental Code of Conduct to address areas that are not covered in the APA Code of Ethics. These latest Rules were adopted on March 18, 2004 and became effective April 7, 2004.

boundaries. Another excellent reference, which is also more of a practical handbook rather than a formal textbook, is provided in Pope and Vasquez's (1998) *Ethics in Psychotherapy and Counseling: A Practical Guide for Psychologists*. Pope and Vasquez address a wide array of ethical topics from a conservative perspective. Kenneth Pope also provides an extensive review of other ethics articles and practical resources at http://www.kspope.com/index.php.

Providing a rebuttal to the conventional wisdom of the slippery slope argument, Lazarus and Zur's (2002) *Dual Relationships and Psychotherapy* is creative and challenging in its discussion of the dual relationships in psychotherapy. With a total of 31 chapters written by contributing authors ranging from psychologists and psychiatrists to law professors and trial lawyers, Lazarus and Zur argue in favor of the value of nonsexual dual relationships in psychotherapy. The book contains over two dozen chapters on a variety of dual relationships that arise in bartering arrangements, deaf communities, multicultural communities, church settings, military protocol, feminist therapy, and student counseling centers. In my opinion, "The contributing authors are to be commended for their courage in challenging orthodox viewpoints and offering alternative opinions that will promote meaningful discussion of dual relationships in psychotherapy" (Doverspike, 2004a, p. 211).

Providing the type of practical guidelines that clinicians need when faced with ethical dilemmas involving dual relationships, Ebert (2006) provides a blend of ethical and legal considerations in *Multiple Relationships and Conflict of Interest for Mental Health Professionals: A Conservative Psycholegal Approach*. Ebert offers a series of decision-making rules that address a variety of situations ranging from social contacts with clients to ethical no-brainers such as insider trading and real estate transactions. The book is filled with case examples ranging from the mundane to the bizarre, including a section on the obvious hazards of "hot-tubbing" with clients. With many of the cases taken from public records of licensing board complaints and malpractice lawsuits, Ebert's case examples illustrate how truth is indeed stranger than fiction. In the broad array of approaches to dual relationships, ranging from the liberal to the conservative ends of the continuum, Ebert's psycholegal book should be placed clearly on the right side of the shelf.

With an emphasis on practical guidelines, Younggren (2002a) provides a useful discussion regarding ethical decision making and dual relationships. When considering engaging in a dual relationship with a client, ask yourself the following questions that are recommended by Younggren:

- Is the dual relationship necessary?
- Is the dual relationship exploitive?
- Whom does the dual relationship benefit?
- Is there a risk that the dual relationship could damage the patient?
- Is there a risk that the dual relationship could disrupt the therapeutic relationship?
- Are you being objective in your evaluation of this matter?

Once a therapist has addressed the previous questions, which are designed to protect the interests of the client, Younggren recommends that the therapist shift into a risk-management mode by asking the following questions: First, did the client give informed consent regarding the risks of engaging in the dual relationship? Second, have you adequately documented your decision-making process (including the client's informed consent) in the treatment records?

In summary, a brief review of the literature on dual relationships reveals a diversity of opinions ranging from the staunchly conservative to the creatively liberal. These trends in the field of ethics and dual relationships have an implication for the contemporary psychotherapist: If you are too conservative, consider loosening up a bit; if you are too liberal, consider tightening up a bit. Whatever your position, consider the merits of other positions, because the most reasonable position may lie somewhere between the ends of the continuum.

Role-Blending

Role-blending involves having two or more professional roles with the same person, usually at the same time. Role-blending involves two professional roles, whereas dual relationships involve one role that is professional and another role that is usually nonprofessional (e.g., social, financial, political). In other words, role-blending involves a specific type of dual relationship in which both roles are professional. Some professional roles involve an inherent duality, such as when educators serve not only as instructors and teachers but also as supervisors and mentors, sometimes even engaging in social roles for the purpose of benefiting their students. Although supervision and psychotherapy are two completely different processes, they also share some common aspects such as a power differential, self-disclosure, and a focus on relational dynamics. For example, there are times when a supervisor may engage in some role-blending by assisting a supervisee in identifying ways that his or her personal dynamics are blocking his or her ability to work effectively with clients. This blending of the roles of supervisor and therapeutic agent is different from a purely psychotherapeutic role because the supervisor keeps the focus in the present, on the client, and on the treatment.

There are also some clinical roles that involve an inherent duality, such as when psychologists work for managed care organizations (MCO) or when professional counselors work for community service boards. In managed care environments, the provider's dual roles involve a primary fiduciary duty to the patient counterbalanced with the provider's contractual agreement with the MCO, which may involve decisions that are not always in the best interests of the patient. In community service agencies, professional counselors may be required to perform multiple roles such as working as both a counselor and a case manager. G. Corey et al. (2007, p. 492) describe several roles that counselors may be required to perform in community settings, including the roles of advisor, advocate, consultant, change agent, facilitator of indigenous support systems, and facilitator of indigenous healing systems. From a risk-management perspective, where there are multiple roles, there are multiple opportunities for role-blending, blurring, and confusion.

Although blending of some roles is ethical and inevitable, blending of other roles is always unethical and indefensible. Examples of ethical role-blending might involve serving both as a teacher and a clinical supervisor in a university counseling center, or serving as a counselor and a case manager at a community service board or mental health center. Examples of unethical role-blending might involve serving as a psychotherapist and engaging in a joint venture as a business partner, or serving as a clinical supervisor and a psychotherapist of the supervisee. One area of unethical role-blending that continues to receive increased scrutiny involves the irreconcilable conflict between therapeutic and forensic roles (Greenberg & Shuman, 1997; Harris, 2004; Younggren, 2006).

The problem with any role-blending is that it can create conflicts of interest and a loss of objectivity. Role-blending calls for vigilance on the part of the professional to ensure that exploitation does not occur. Role-blending must be managed carefully, collaboratively, and consultatively in order to increase the benefits of the person being served and in order to reduce the risk of harm or exploitation. In other words, be careful, collaborate to determine the client's best interests, and consult with a colleague to avoid unintentional role blurring or confusion.

Conflicts of Interest

In plain English, role-blending and dual roles involve concepts that clients may more readily understand as *conflicts of interest*, a term that is often more easily used when discussing the potential problems of engaging in dual roles with clients. APA (2002) Ethical Standard 3.06 (Conflict of Interest) states, "Psychologists refrain from taking on a professional role when personal, scientific, professional, legal, financial, or other interests or relationships could reasonably be expected to (1) impair their objectivity, competence, or effectiveness in performing their functions as psychologists or (2) expose the person or organization with whom the professional relationship exists to harm or exploitation" (p. 1065).

In my own consultations with colleagues, I often use the simple test of a "conflicts check" to improve ethical vision by assessing whether a contemplated role change will pass the ethical test. Based on APA Ethical Standard 3.06, a conflicts check includes five basic questions, listed in order from the most sensitive to the least sensitive screening criteria. When you are operating in a professional role (e.g., psychotherapist, counselor, employer, supervisor, researcher, teacher) and you are contemplating role-blending or boundary crossing, consider asking yourself these five questions:

- Is there a chance of *loss of effectiveness* of the professional? If yes, then stop. If no, then proceed to the next step.
- Is there a chance of *loss of objectivity* of the professional? If yes, then stop. If no, then proceed to the next step.
- Is there a chance of *loss of competence* of the professional? If yes, then stop. If no, then proceed to the next step.
- Is there a chance of *risk of exploitation* of the client? If yes, then stop. If no, then proceed to the next step.
- Is there a chance of *risk of harm* to the client? If yes, then stop. If no, then proceed with caution after collaborating to determine the client's best interests and consulting with a colleague to identify any ethical blind spots.

Incidental Encounters

Incidental encounters refer to chance encounters between therapist and client outside the professional setting. Incidental encounters with current or former clients may occur randomly or by chance in a variety of settings, such as a grocery store, shopping mall, public ceremony, religious service, 12-step meeting, and so forth. Incidental encounters are essentially brief, unforeseeable concurrent dual roles. However, because the professional does not necessarily step out of the primary professional role, incidental encounters are not the same as dual relationships.

Many therapists are reluctant to even acknowledge clients outside the professional setting. According to Hyman (2002, p. 351), "the common stance, whether intentional of not, seems to be avoidance of full human contact (i.e., not approaching the client, not initiating a conversation) during the encounters and detailed analysis of the interaction during subsequent therapy sessions." Nevertheless, incidental encounters with current psychotherapy clients can be grist for the therapeutic mill in the client's next session.

Hybrid Relationships

Hybrid relationship is a term that can be applied to a dual relationship that combines professional and social roles. For the enlightenment of conservative therapists, a hybrid relationship refers to a relationship that is "partly friendship and partly professional" (Golden, 2002, p. 414). Unlike role-blending, which combines two professional roles (e.g., therapist and case manager), a so-called hybrid relationship combines a professional role and a social role. The following brief excerpt gives an example of a therapist's reflections of a hybrid relationship in which a professional relationship seems to morph into a social relationship with a client:

> Our conversations began straying beyond the strictly therapeutic, as we talked about mundane life and I started participating more, inaugurating a transition away from the one-sidedness of psychotherapy. I was enjoying her company, and we began to shift into a "hybrid" relationship, one that was partly friendship and partly professional. Just after 2 years from when we met, our professional relationship came to an official end. . . . (Golden, 2002, p. 414)

Although such a relationship can be classified as a foreseeable (i.e., contemplated) concurrent dual relationship based on the classification scheme in Table 1 (p. 50), the idea of a so-called hybrid relationship seems to define deviance downward by giving new meaning to the concept of blurred boundaries. In my opinion, relationships that are partly professional and partly friendship are in reality neither professional nor friendly (Doverspike, 2004a).

RISK FACTORS
AND UNHEALTHY BOUNDARIES

Stealth Dilemmas

Stealth dilemmas are essentially ethical dilemmas that sneak up on therapists. Some therapists do not see the headlights of an approaching conflict of interest even though their feet have been run over by them in the past. The dilemmas that sneak up on some therapists are the ethical dilemmas that are obvious to more vigilant therapists. Dilemmas that are obvious are dilemmas that are preventable by vigilant therapists. The best way to avoid stealth dilemmas is through cultivating a sense of ethical self-awareness, using informed consent to prevent ethical problems before they arise, managing boundaries appropriately from the outset, recognizing the first step toward the slippery slope, and consulting with colleagues to identify ethical blind spots.

Ethical Blind Spots

Ethical blind spots are areas of poor vision in which there is some lack of knowledge or lack of awareness. Blind spots can be related to deficits in technical competence, including lack of knowledge (i.e., ignorance or misinformation) as well as deficits in emotional competence (i.e., psychological factors such as denial, narcissism, and countertransference). Just as ethical blind spots are one of the most dangerous ways to get on the slippery slope, improving one's ethical vision is one of the best ways to see the slopes before stepping onto them. Ethical vision can be improved through continuing ethical education and developing a sense of ethical self-awareness. Trusted methods of improving ethical vision involve clinical supervision, personal psychotherapy, continuing education, and ongoing consultation.

Early Warning Signs

Early warning signs, which are sometimes called red flags, are signs of unhealthy boundaries in the therapeutic relationships. These include dynamics such as overinvolvement or overidentification with the client, feeling overly responsible for the client's progress, being manipulated by the client's demands, and responding inappropriately to personal questions by the client. A factor underlying all of these dynamics is denial, or simply not noticing boundary slippage by the therapist or boundary intrusion by the client. Early warning signs signal the need for clinical supervision, personal psychotherapy, continuing education, and ongoing consultation.

Slippery Slope Phenomena

Slippery slope phenomena essentially involve the subtle transition from boundary crossings to boundary violations. Although boundary crossings are not inherently unethical, the problem with boundary crossings is that they can place a therapist on a slippery slope. The slippery slope argument is based on the premise that boundary crossings of therapists will "inevitably lead to a progressive deterioration of ethical behavior" (G. Corey et al., 2007, p. 270) down a slope that will eventually result in boundary violations. One postulate of the slippery slope argument is that if psychotherapists do not adhere to rigid standards, their behavior may foster relationships that are sexual or otherwise harmful to clients (Gabbard, 1994). The first step down the slippery slope begins with a boundary crossing. To avoid going down the slippery slope, therapists are advised to manage boundaries conservatively, have a therapeutic rationale for every boundary crossing, and question behaviors that are inconsistent with their theoretical approach (Pope, Sonne, & Holroyd, 1993; D. Smith & Fitzpatrick, 1995).

Although there seems to be little controversy among ethicists regarding the slippery slope argument as it relates to sexualized boundary violations, there has been an ongoing debate regarding the slippery slope hypothesis as it relates to nonsexual boundary crossings. On the one hand, there has been a traditional consensus of opinion among conservative ethicists (e.g., Pope & Vasquez, 1991, 1998) that therapists who push nonsexual boundaries are more likely to become sexually involved with clients. On the other hand, there has been an opinion among more liberal ethicists (e.g., Lazarus, 2001; Lazarus & Zur, 2002) that nonsexual boundary crossings do not necessarily lead to sexual boundary violations. As Lazarus (2001) states, "Too many therapists see only a negative and hazardous side to all dual relationships. They claim that harm is inevitable, faulty clinical judgments will ensue, and in terms of risk management, great dangers lurk behind every corner" (p. 16).

Between the extremes of the conservative and liberal positions, there is also the more moderate position (e.g., Doverspike, 2004a) that nonsexual boundary crossings may lead to nonsexual boundary violations. The main reason to avoid the slippery slope of nonsexual boundary crossings is because they can *inadvertently* lead to nonsexual boundary violations. The ethical drift involved in boundary blurring is often seen in troubled therapists who confess that their initial decisions to cross boundaries eventually led to their next logical steps in the progression of a downward spiral of increasingly harmful boundary violations, at which point the initial boundary crossing that started the chain of events is barely visible from the event horizon. Nonsexual boundary violations alone are often enough to harm clients. Because the potential for harm may not always be foreseeable, the best way to avoid harm to the client is to stay off the slope in the first place. In other words, the best way to avoid the risk of boundary violations is to avoid boundary crossings.

SEXUAL IMPROPRIETY

A colleague on a state ethics committee once said that the single best way to avoid the most serious of ethics complaints was to "never have sex with a client." One might add, "or a former client." This advice may seem so obvious that it doesn't need repeating, yet sexual misconduct represents the most serious ethical breach of our profession. Indeed, sexual misconduct is generally considered the most egregious unethical behavior, regardless of one's professional identity or theoretical orientation (Borys & Pope, 1989). Sexual impropriety accounts for approximately half of the costs of malpractice cases and over 20% of the total number of claims (Pope, 1989a; Pope & Vasquez, 1991; Stromberg & Dellinger, 1993). In an effort to reduce such claims, most professional liability insurance policies exclude coverage of sexual impropriety. Although such policies typically provide coverage for the defense of so-called "sex claims," there may be no coverage in the event that sexual misconduct is admitted or proven. The situation can become much more complex if the sexual misconduct is admitted or proven on the part of a psychologist's employee or supervisee who is covered under the psychologist's insurance policy.

Sexual misconduct was one of the most frequent reasons for licensing board disciplinary actions for psychologists from 1983 to 2001 (K. Kirkland et al., 2004). Although many studies have focused on psychologists, the only national study using the same survey instrument during the same time period with respondents from three major mental health professions found *no significant difference* among the rates at which psychiatrists, psychologists, and social workers acknowledged engaging in sex with their patients (Borys & Pope, 1989). Borys and Pope reported that 0.5% of their respondents acknowledged having engaged in sexual activity with a current client, and 3.9% of the respondents acknowledged having engaged in sexual activity with a client after termination of professional services.

Gabbard and Pope (1988) have documented the many harmful effects of "professional incest." In almost every complaint of sexual misconduct, there are also other boundary violations as well. Even when allegations of sexual misconduct cannot be proven, allegations of boundary violations can almost always be proven. When boundary violations begin to occur, a clinician may start sliding down the slippery slope toward sexual misconduct. Although a mandatory ethical obligation would be to "never have sex with a client," a more aspirational standard would be to "maintain clear boundaries with clients." By way of analogy, everyone knows that a driver shouldn't fall asleep at the wheel while driving. Although some people do fall asleep, the warning line should not be "don't fall asleep at the wheel," but rather "don't drive when you are tired."

What's the difference between a psychiatrist and psychologist? A psychiatric colleague once joked to me that the difference was that psychologists "have to wait 2 years before having sex with their patients." Although his comment reflected a distorted view of the American Psychological Association standard, my psychiatric colleague and I agreed that "once a patient, *always* a patient." In other words, there is no such thing as a "former patient." Some ethicists "believe the statement 'Once a client, always a client' is a dogmatic pronouncement that should be subject to discussion" (G. Corey et al., 2007, p. 304). However, because APA 2002 Ethical Standard 10.07 (Therapy With Former Sexual Partners) states that "Psychologists do not accept as therapy clients/patients persons with whom they have engaged in sexual intimacies" (p. 1073), then having a sexual relationship with a former client (even after a substantial time lapse) would effectively prevent the former client from being able to return to psychotherapy with the same therapist at a later time. Interestingly, the ACA (2005) *Code of Ethics* does not specifically prohibit counselors from accepting as therapy clients those persons with whom the counselor has previously engaged in sexual intimacies, although the ACA *Code of Ethics** does advise counselors to avoid supervising those persons whom

---

* Reprinted from the 2005 *ACA Code of Ethics.* Copyright © 2005 by the American Counseling Association. Reprinted with permission. No further reproduction authorized without written permission from the American Counseling Association.

the counselor has had as romantic partners or friends. ACA (2005) Section F.3.d (Close Relatives and Friends) states, "Counseling supervisors avoid accepting close relatives, romantic partners, or friends as supervisees." Counselors striving for excellence in maintaining integrity in boundaries would be advised to apply this same standard to all clients being considered for counseling or psychotherapy. Lest this prohibition be considered another "dogmatic pronouncement," counselors should avoid accepting close relatives, romantic partners, or friends as clients for counseling and psychotherapy.

In reviewing the results of their national survey of psychiatrists' attitudes concerning sexual intimacies with their clients, Herman et al. (1987) point out that the concept of a so-called "posttermination waiting period" before sexual intimacies are initiated is naïve because it disregards both the continued inequity of roles of the therapist and former client, and it ignores the "timelessness of unconscious processes" (p. 168). In making observations about psychotherapists' views of their own personal therapy, Buckley, Karasu, and Charles (1981) observe, "Analysis of the data also revealed that thoughts about the therapist reach a peak during the 5-10 year period following treatment. . . . All of the respondents in the 5-10 year period following therapy reported experiencing thoughts of returning to analysis or therapy. This would seem to be a critical time in the post-therapeutic development" (p. 304). It is not only the length of time that renders posttherapeutic sexual relations unethical, it is the nature of the original professional relationship itself. In describing posttherapeutic sexual relationships as a form of professional incest, Brodsky (as cited in Sanders, 1997, p. 89) observes, "Father-daughter incest does not become acceptable one year after the daughter has left home. No matter how the therapy contract ends, the imbalance of power of the initial interactions can never be erased."

Posttherapeutic professional incest is ethically prohibited in the field of psychiatry. *The Principles of Medical Ethics With Annotations Especially Applicable to Psychiatry* (American Psychiatric Association, 2001) includes the following unequivocal statement: "Sexual activity with a current or former patient is unethical" (§ 2.1). Legislatively oriented clinicians should be reminded of the leadership provided by Florida psychologists with respect to prohibition of posttherapeutic sexual relationships and protection of the posttherapeutic professional relationship. State of Florida Chapter 21U-15.004 once stated, "For purposes of determining the existence of sexual misconduct as defined herein, the psychologist-client relationship is deemed to continue in perpetuity." As later amended, Chapter 64B19-16.003 of the Florida

Administrative Code for Psychologists (2001) states, "The mere passage of time since the client's last visit to the psychologist is not solely determinative of whether or not the psychologist-client relationship has been terminated." It may be helpful to remember that mental health professionals have other continuing responsibilities and obligations to clients (e.g., maintaining confidentiality and protecting privilege) that are not affected by the "passage of time after termination" (Gabbard & Pope, 1988, p. 23). Because a client has the right to renew a professional relationship in the future, one must assume that a professional relationship continues to exist as long as the client assumes that it does, regardless of the amount of time that has elapsed in the interim (Gottlieb, 1993).

Regarding the matter of sexual relationships with former clients, the National Association of Social Workers (NASW) takes Gottlieb's (1993) recommendation seriously. Section 1.09.c. of the NASW (1999) *Code of Ethics* states, "Social workers should not engage in sexual activities or sexual conduct with former clients because of the potential for harm to the client." With a policy that is more liberal than NASW and more conservative than APA, the ACA (2005) has shifted from a 2-year to a 5-year posttermination statute. Section A.5.b. (Former Clients) of the ACA *Code of Ethics* states, "Sexual or romantic counselor-client interactions or relationships with former clients, their romantic partners, or their family members are prohibited for a period of 5 years following the last professional contact." Psychologists striving for excellence in preserving the sanctity of the posttherapeutic relationship would be advised to apply the ACA standard or, even better, to adopt the NASW standard which clearly prohibits posttherapeutic sexual contact with former clients.

It may be helpful to clarify a common misunderstanding regarding the so-called posttherapeutic "waiting period." Some psychologists seem to believe that APA (2002) Ethical Standard 10.08 (Sexual Intimacies With Former Therapy Clients/Patients) gives a "green light" to sexual involvement with former clients 2 years after the termination of psychotherapy. This is *not* true. APA Ethical Standard 10.08(b) states that "Psychologists who engage in such activity after the two years following cessation or termination of therapy and of having no sexual contact with the former client/patient bear the burden of demonstrating that there has been no exploitation" of the former client (p. 1073). The prototype given in the APA debates over this section of the code deals with the hypothetical psychologist who might meet a former client in a social situation many years after having conducted one session of career counseling with the person. Although scenarios of such "unusual circumstances" might be possible, they are indeed rare and clinicians can get themselves into trouble if they start thinking of clients as potential romantic partners. Although the 2-year period has been described as a "flashing red light," it should be viewed as a stop sign on a dead-end street.

The prohibition of sexualized dual relationships may also extend to persons with whom the client has "an affectionate personal relationship" (Pope, 1986, p. 25). At least one version of the *Psychologist's Professional Liability Policy* administered by the American Professional Agency and issued by the American Home Assurance Company (AHAC; 1990) has included special provisions that limit coverage for any claims of sexual involvement "with or to any former or current patient or client of any Insured, or with or to any relative of or member of the same household as any said patient or client, or with or to any person with whom the patient or client or relative has an affectionate personal relationship" (p. 3). As emphasized by Pope (1986), actual erotic, physical contact need not be present because included in the provisions of the AHAC policy is any "attempt threat or proposal thereof" (p. 25). Pope further pointed out that proposals or attempts at erotic, physical contact need not actually occur but need only be "alleged at any time" (p. 25). Clearly, the rule of thumb is to avoid even the *appearance* of impropriety, which means setting clear limits and maintaining firm boundaries from the first session onward.

SPECIAL CONSIDERATIONS

Therapist Self-Disclosure

Depending on one's theoretical perspective, a therapist's use of self-disclosure as a therapeutic technique may range from the traditional psychoanalytic rule of abstinence (Greenson, 1967; Hall, 1998) to the humanistic process of transparency (Jourard, 1971). In terms of content, therapist self-disclosure can range from the purely professional to the pruriently personal. In terms of the focus of the disclosure, the continuum can range from client-oriented to therapist-oriented disclosures. In terms of the degree of intimacy of a therapist's self-disclosure, the continuum can vary from low to high. For example, a low-intimacy, therapist-oriented therapist disclosure of facts and credentials might simply involve the therapist providing information about his or her education, training, or theoretical orientation. A low-intimacy, client-oriented therapist disclosure might involve approval or reassurance, such as sharing information about a situation similar to the client's situation. At higher levels of intimacy, disclosures might involve sharing of the therapist's feelings (e.g., such as using specific words to describe the therapist's emotional experiences), cognitive insights (e.g., such as describing lessons learned about the underlying dynamics of a situation), or adaptive behavioral strategies (e.g., describing coping strategies or actions the therapist found useful in dealing with a similar situation). Of course, this classification scheme is not meant to imply that any of the preceding types of therapist disclosures are ethical or unethical, but simply to clarify the conceptual differences among various types of therapist self-disclosures. Table 2 (below) illustrates four types of therapist disclosures based on the dimensions of content of disclosure (client-oriented vs. therapist-oriented) and degree of intimacy (low intimacy vs. high intimacy).

Table 2: Examples of Types of Therapist Disclosures

	Client-Oriented	**Therapist-Oriented**
Low Intimacy	Low-intimacy client-oriented	Low-intimacy therapist-oriented
High Intimacy	High-intimacy client-oriented	High-intimacy therapist-oriented

Table 2 depicts four types of therapist self-disclosures, each of which is illustrated by one of the following examples: A *low-intimacy client-oriented* disclosure might involve a therapist expressing approval, encouragement, or reassurance to a client, whereas a *low-intimacy therapist-oriented* disclosure might involve a therapist stating facts about his or her theoretical approach, credentials, education, or training. A *high-intimacy client-oriented* disclosure might involve a therapist sharing feelings with the client or sharing strategies that the therapist has used to surmount challenges in his or her own life, whereas a *high-intimacy therapist-oriented* disclosure might involve a therapist sharing highly personal information about the therapist's own functioning in relationships. This method of classifying special events is not meant to imply that any of the previous types of therapist self-disclosures is ethical or unethical, but simply to clarify the differences between the types.

The previous classification is not meant to imply that therapist self-disclosure is simply a dichotomous concept that can be neatly divided into two categories. In reality, self-disclosure is a multidimensional concept that includes various dimensions such as level of intimacy that, for example, may occur on a continuum ranging from low intimacy to high intimacy and everything in between. Neither the previous classification nor the empirical surveys of self-disclosure (e.g., Gibson & Pope, 1993; Pope et al., 1987) address other forms of therapist disclosure such as subtle voice inflection, body language, and eye contact. The nonverbal behavior and body language of the therapist, especially including differential eye contact, can give clients a subtle but powerful indication of the therapist's values as well as how the therapist is affected by the client. For example, a marital therapist may communicate a powerful message when he or she looks at a husband when asking questions about family finances or when the therapist looks at a wife when asking about child-rearing practices, or vice versa. In addition, therapist disclosure may also occur in subtle but significant ways by jewelry worn by the therapist (e.g., a cross, crucifix, crescent, or Star of David), various photos displayed in the office (e.g., family, friends, and significant others), or even office furnishings (e.g., Asian art, African artifacts, Native American pottery) that communicate cultural information. Although these other forms of therapist disclosure may be subtler than verbal self-disclosure, they may reveal just as much information about the therapist's values, feelings, and attitudes toward the client and others.

A national survey of professional psychologists revealed that 38.6% of professional psychologists reported sometimes "using self-disclosure as a therapeutic technique" and 43.0% respondents agreed that "using self-disclosure as a therapeutic technique" was ethical "under many circumstances" (Pope et al., 1987, p. 995). A national survey of certified counselors indicated that 92% of the participants reported that "using self-disclosure as a counseling technique" was ethical, although the survey did not report how often the participants engaged in the behavior of using self-disclosure (Gibson & Pope, 1993, p. 332). A similar national survey was conducted with Christian counselors, as identified by membership in the American Association of Christian Counselors (AACC), with an additional data analysis for those AACC members who were also members of the Christian Association for Psychological Studies (CAPS). The survey of AACC and CAPS members indicated that 45% of the total sample and 52% of CAPS respondents reported sometimes "using self-disclosure as a therapy technique" and 40% of the total sample and 42% of the CAPS respondents agreed that "using self-disclosure as a therapy technique" was ethical "under many circumstances" (McMinn, Meek, & McRay, 1997, p. 29).

In my own practice of psychotherapy and ethics consultations, I find myself asking the same questions that I ask my supervisees to ask when working with their clients.

When considering making a self-disclosure to a client, ask yourself these questions:

- Is the contemplated self-disclosure consistent with your theoretical orientation? If self-disclosure is not consistent with your theoretical orientation, then don't self-disclose.
- If self-disclosure is consistent with your theoretical orientation, then is self-disclosure part of your treatment plan with a particular client? If it is not part of your treatment plan, then don't self-disclose.
- If self-disclosure is part of your treatment plan, then is there a way to accomplish the same treatment objective without using self-disclosure? If there is another way to accomplish the objective, then consider using less self-disclosing options first.
- How well are you managing clear boundaries and maintaining therapeutic neutrality? When in the process of therapy is the self-disclosure occurring? What are your motivations for self-disclosing? If you are already having trouble managing boundaries and maintaining neutrality, then don't self-disclose.
- How intact are the client's boundaries, reality testing abilities, psychological strengths, and levels of functioning? In other words, are there any clinical contraindications regarding the use of self-disclosure? Are there any indications that the client might sexualize or otherwise misinterpret the self-disclosure? If the client has weak ego boundaries or distorted perceptions of reality, then consider that likelihood that your self-disclosure could result in confusion, misinterpretations, or distortion on the part of your client.
- What are the multicultural implications of the self-disclosure? In other words, what is the significance of the disclosure in terms of the client's age, sex, race, ethnicity, religion, national origin, indigenous heritage, or sexual orientation?
- Where does the contemplated self-disclosure fit on the continuum of intimate to nonintimate information? If the self-disclosure

involves nonintimate information (e.g., policies, procedures, and credentials), then self-disclosure is more likely to be appropriate. If the self-disclosure involves more personal information (e.g., social activities, marital functioning, personal feelings), then consider all the other options before using self-disclosure.

• How well can you defend your disclosure to your professional peers? Think how you would feel if you saw your self-disclosure published in licensing board proceedings, in an ethics article on boundaries, or in a court transcript of a professional liability suit.

• What is in the client's best interest?

The Use of Touch

Although there is a consensus of opinion that erotic and sexual forms of touch are unethical in counseling and psychotherapy (Borys & Pope, 1989), some forms of nonerotic touch are considered acceptable. Whether a therapist uses touch may depend in part on the therapist's theoretical orientation. Some clinicians oppose any form of physical contact with clients on the grounds that it will promote dependency or interfere with the transference relationship. From a risk-management perspective, other therapists avoid the use of touch because it can be sexualized or otherwise misinterpreted by a client. Other clinicians (e.g., Rabinowitz, 1991) argue that appropriate touching can foster self-exploration, increase verbal interaction, increase the client's perception of the expertness of the counselor, and can produce more positive attitudes toward the counseling process.

Touch may be roughly classified along a continuum ranging from clearly acceptable to clearly unacceptable forms of touch, with most forms of touch falling in between these two extremes. There is a general consensus of opinion that some forms of touch are clearly unacceptable (Borys & Pope, 1989; Pope et al., 1987). Inappropriate forms of touch would include sexual or romantic touches as well as hostile, punishing, violent, or other offensive forms of touch (e.g., pushing or hitting a client). On the other hand, it may be appropriate to use defensive forms of touch to prevent a client from harming himself or herself, to prevent someone from hurting another person, or as a form of self-defense with respect to a violent patient.

Perhaps the most acceptable forms of touch are the ritualistic or socially accepted gestures for greeting. A national survey of professional psychologists revealed that a total of 93.8% of professional psychologists reported sometimes, fairly often, or very often "offering or accepting a handshake from client." In terms of ethicality of the behavior, 3.3% of professional psychologist respondents agreed that "offering or accepting a handshake from a client" was "sometimes" ethical, 21.7% of the respondents agreed that "offering or accepting a handshake from client" was ethical "under many circumstances," and an additional 71.9% reported that "unquestionably yes" (ethical) for this item (Pope et al., 1987, p. 997). In other words, a total of 96.9% percent of psychologist respondents agreed that "offering or accepting a handshake from client" was at least sometimes acceptable. In contrast, only 4.6% of psychologists reported that they never or rarely shook hands with clients. A national survey of certified counselors indicated that 99% of the participants reported that "offering or accepting a handshake from client" was ethical, although the survey did not report how often the participants engaged in the behavior of using self-disclosure (Gibson & Pope, 1993, p. 333). However, from a multicultural perspective it is important to remember that a behavior as seemingly benign as offering a handshake may violate the norms and customs of some cultural and religious groups.

Another generally acceptable form of touch includes the use of touch based on one's theoretical orientation or treatment procedures, such as the use of touch as a conversation marker, as a hypnotic induction procedure, or as an "anchor" in neurolinguistic programming (Dilts, 1983; Lankton, 1980). Other forms of acceptable touch include consolation touch, reassuring touch, playful touch, grounding or reorienting touch, task-oriented touch, instructional or modeling touch, celebratory or congratulatory touch, or inadvertent touch. Somewhere in the middle of the continuum of acceptable and unacceptable forms of touch are those techniques that are somewhat more controversial, such as the use of touch as an experiential touch (e.g., psychodrama), as a form of corrective emotional experience (e.g., cradling), or as a form of process-oriented Rolfing (Rolf, 1989).

Hugging is a form of touch that has been subject to considerable discussion. Rabinowitz (1991) states, "It may be safer for a hug to occur in group therapy rather than in individual counseling because there are witnesses to the context of the touching in a group, leaving less room for misinterpretation" (p. 576). Pope et al. (1987) reported that 29.8% of professional psychologists reported sometimes "hugging a client" and 45.5% respondents agreed that "hugging a client" was ethical "under many circumstances" (p. 995). A national survey of certified counselors indicated that 86% of the participants reported that "hugging a client" was ethical, although the survey did not report how often the participants engaged in the behavior (Gibson & Pope, 1993, p. 332). A national survey of Christian counselors, as identified by membership in AACC (with additional data analysis for those who were also CAPS members) indicated that 34% of the total sample and 39% of CAPS respondents reported sometimes "hugging a client" and 36% of the total sample and 35% of the CAPS respondents agreed that "hugging a client" was ethical "under many circumstances" (McMinn et al., 1997, p. 28).

Bennett et al. (1990) offer some guidelines regarding the nonerotic use of touch with psychotherapy clients. Ask yourself how well you know the client, whether touch is appropriate under the specific circumstances, and whether the touch is indicated in a particular situation. Bennett et al. point out that the most important question from a risk-management perspective involves whether the touch can be misinterpreted by the client (or the client's family) as a sexual overtone.

When considering the therapeutic use of nonerotic forms of touch such as the therapeutic use of touch or the occasional hug, ask yourself these questions:

- Is there an institutional policy regarding the use of touch? If an institutional policy forbids the use of touch (such as hugging a patient in a psychiatric hospital or hugging an inmate in a corrections facility), then don't touch.
- Is the use of touch consistent with your theoretical orientation? If the use of touch is not consistent with your theoretical orientation, then don't touch.
- If the use of touch is consistent with your theoretical orientation, then is it part of your treatment plan with a particular client? If it is not part of your treatment plan, then don't touch.
- If the use of touch is part of your treatment plan, then is there a way to accomplish the same treatment objective without using touch? If there is another way to accomplish the objective, then consider using other methods first.
- How well are you managing clear boundaries and maintaining therapeutic neutrality? When in the process of therapy is the use of touch occurring? What are your motivations for using touch? If you are already having trouble managing boundaries, then don't touch.
- How intact are the client's ego boundaries, reality testing abilities, psychological strengths, and levels of functioning? In other words, are there any clinical contraindications regarding the use of touch? Are there any indications that the client might sexualize or

otherwise misinterpret the touch? If the client has weak ego boundaries or distorted perceptions of reality, then consider the likelihood that touch could result in confusion, misinterpretations, or distortions on the part of the client.

- What are the multicultural implications of using touch? In other words, what is the significance of the use of touch in terms of the client's age, sex, race, ethnicity, religion, national origin, indigenous heritage, or sexual orientation?
- Are there others present when you use touch? In general, when there are witnesses present (such as in a group therapy situation), the touch is less likely to be misinterpreted by the client and others.
- How well can you defend your use of touch to your professional peers? Think how you would feel if you saw a picture of yourself published in a newspaper depicting you touching your client.
- What is in the client's best interest?

Bartering for Services

Bartering involves exchanging professional services for nonmonetary goods or services. Although the most conservative position is simply not to barter at all, some ethicists take a more liberal view toward bartering. For example, G. Corey et al. (2007) state, "Bartering is an example of a dual relationship that we think allows some room for practitioners, in collaboration with their clients, to use good judgment and consider the cultural context in the situation" (pp. 280-281). Hill (1999) discusses bartering as a legitimate way of helping out a poor but needy person. Thomas (2002) describes bartering as "a relatively dignified way for the patient to compensate the therapist for professional work" (p. 394). Bartering for services is not prohibited by the Ethics Code of any mental health profession, yet it is often so highly problematic that it deserves special consideration. Bartering is not necessarily unethical, but it may lead to ethical problems. From a risk-management perspective, particularly because professionals always have the option of providing some services pro bono, bartering should probably be used as a last resort.

When considering whether or not to accept goods rather than money in exchange for services, Pope et al. (1987) reported that only 6.4% of professional psychologists reported sometimes "accepting goods (rather than money) as payment" and only 18.2% of respondents agreed that "accepting goods (rather than money) as payment" was ethical "under many circumstances" (p. 995). Similarly, Pope et al. reported that only

3.5% of professional psychologists reported sometimes "accepting services from a client in lieu of fee" and only 16.0% of respondents agreed that "accepting services from a client in lieu of fee" was ethical "under many circumstances" (p. 995). A national survey of certified counselors indicated that 63% of the participants reported that "accepting goods (rather than money) as payment" was ethical, and 53% of the participants reported that "accepting services from a client in lieu of fee" was ethical (Gibson & Pope, 1993, p. 332). Gibson and Pope's study did not address the frequency of occurrence of these behaviors. These studies suggest that counselors report somewhat more permissive attitudes toward bartering than do psychologists, and that counselors and psychologists view accepting goods (rather than money) as somewhat more ethical than accepting services (rather than money) as payment for professional services. However, there is not strong evidence that either professional group strongly supports the use of either type of bartering.

In my experience in adjudicating ethics complaints, some of the most serious boundary violations can often be traced back to what could have been initially viewed as simple bartering arrangements. Does anyone need to be reminded that one of the original licensing board complaints that sparked the debate on nonsexual dual relationships over 2 decades ago involved a therapist who bartered for services with a client? When the client complained to the California Board of Psychology (*In the Matter of the Accusation Against Leon Jerome Oziel, Ph.D.*, 1986), it was determined that the client had paid more than $1,000 dollars per hour for therapy when the hours of therapy were compared to the number of hours that the client had provided in landscaping of the psychologist's home. What was reasonable to Dr. Oziel was not reasonable to his state licensing board. Keep in mind that if the client perceives harm or exploitation associated with a bartering arrangement, the burden of proof will rest on the psychologist to demonstrate that the prospective bartering arrangement could not reasonably have been expected to result in harm or exploitation.

Notwithstanding the arguments against bartering, there are some general guidelines that can be used for practitioners who are intent on considering the use of bartering goods and services. Consider bartering only if the client requests it, only if it is not exploitive to the client, and only if it is not clinically contraindicated. When evaluating clinical contraindications, consider factors such as the client's strengths, weaknesses, boundaries, and history of being exploited by others. Bartering should be considered only if it is an accepted cultural practice in the local community. It is important to determine the value of goods or services in a collaborative manner at the outset and to establish a clear, written contract in advance. Consider consultation with a colleague in order to evaluate whether the arrangement will create any risk of a conflict of interest (e.g., using the conflicts checklist described previously in this chapter). Woody (1998) recommends that clinicians minimize any unique financial arrangements. If bartering is used, it is usually better to exchange for goods rather than services. Woody recommends that both the therapist and client should have a signed, written, time-limited agreement.

When considering accepting goods or services rather than money from a client as payment for professional services, ask yourself these questions:

- Is there an institutional policy regarding bartering? If an institutional policy forbids bartering, then don't barter.
- What is the monetary value of the exchange? In general, the greater the monetary value of the exchange, the more likely the risk of perceived harm or exploitation to the client.
- Is bartering consistent with your theoretical orientation? If bartering is not consistent with your theoretical orientation, then don't barter.
- If bartering is consistent with your theoretical orientation, then is it part of your treatment plan with a particular client? If it is not part of your treatment plan, then don't barter.
- If bartering is part of your treatment plan, then is there a way to accomplish the same treatment objective without using bartering? If there is another way to accomplish the objective, then consider using other methods first.
- How well are you managing clear boundaries and maintaining therapeutic neutrality? When in the process of therapy is the use of bartering occurring? What are your motivations for accepting or rejecting a bartering arrangement? If you are already having trouble managing boundaries, then don't barter.
- How intact are the client's ego boundaries, reality testing abilities, psychological strengths, and levels of functioning? In other words, are there any clinical contraindications regarding bartering? Are there any indications that the client might feel exploited or otherwise misinterpret the bartering? If the client has weak ego boundaries or distorted perceptions of reality, then consider the likelihood that bartering could result in confusion, mis-interpretations, or distortions on the part of the client.
- What is the prevailing practice within the local community? In general, the more bartering arrangements are accepted within a

local community, the more likely it will be perceived as an acceptable arrangement.

• What are the multicultural implications of using bartering? In other words, what is the significance of the use of bartering in terms of the client's age, sex, race, ethnicity, religion, national origin, indigenous heritage, or sexual orientation?

• How well can you defend your use of bartering to your professional peers? Think how you would feel if you read a story of yourself describing your bartering arrangement.

• What is in the client's best interest?

Accepting Gifts

No professional code of ethics specifically prohibits accepting a gift from a client, and few professional codes even address the topic of giving or receiving gifts in the therapeutic relationship. Pope et al.'s (1987) survey revealed that 45.0% of professional psychologists reported sometimes "accepting a gift worth less than $5 from a client" and 36.4% respondents agreed that "accepting a gift worth less than $5 from a client" was ethical "under many circumstances" (Pope et al., 1987, p. 997). On the other hand, with regard to a psychologist giving (rather than receiving) a gift, only 8.1% of psychologist participants reported that "giving a gift worth at least $50" was sometimes ethical (p. 996). The monetary value of the gift seems to matter, as evidenced by the finding that only 2.4% of the psychologists responding to the survey reported sometimes "accepting a client's gift worth at least $50" and only 8.6% of the psychologists agreed that "accepting a client's gift worth at least $50" was ethical "under many circumstances" (Pope et al., 1987, p. 995). A national survey of certified counselors indicated that 70% of the participants reported that "accepting a gift worth less than $5 from a client" was ethical (Gibson & Pope, 1993, p. 333), but only 21% of the participants reported that "accepting a client's gift worth at least $50" was ethical (p. 332). On the other hand, only 9% of the certified counselor participants reported that "giving a gift worth at least $50" was ethical.

When considering whether to accept a gift from a client, ask yourself these questions:

• Is there an institutional policy regarding accepting gifts? If an institutional policy forbids accepting gifts, then don't accept gifts.

- What is the monetary value of the gift? In general, the greater the monetary value of the gift, the more likely the risk of perceived harm or exploitation to the client.
- What is the symbolic value of the gift? What is the clinical significance of the client offering the gift?
- Is accepting a gift consistent with your theoretical orientation? If accepting a gift is not consistent with your theoretical orientation, then don't accept it.
- If accepting a gift is consistent with your theoretical orientation, then is it part of your treatment plan with a particular client? If it is not part of your treatment plan, then don't accept it.
- If accepting a gift is part of your treatment plan, then is there a way to accomplish the same treatment objective without accepting the gift? If there is another way to accomplish the objective, then consider other options first.
- How well are you managing clear boundaries and maintaining therapeutic neutrality? When in the process of therapy is the client offering a gift? What are your motivations for accepting or not accepting a gift? If you are already having trouble managing boundaries, then don't accept gifts.
- How intact are the client's ego boundaries, reality testing abilities, psychological strengths, and levels of functioning? In other words, are there any clinical contraindications regarding accepting or not accepting a gift? Are there any indications that the client might feel exploited or otherwise misinterpret your acceptance or rejection of a gift? If the client has weak ego boundaries or distorted perceptions of reality, then consider the likelihood that accepting a gift could result in confusion, misinterpretations, or distortions on the part of the client. On the other hand, consider that rejecting a gift could also result in consequences.
- What is the prevailing practice within the local community? In general, the more that the practice of accepting gifts is considered an acceptable practice within a local community, the more likely it will be perceived as an appropriate arrangement.
- What are the multicultural implications of accepting a gift? In other words, what is the significance of accepting or not accepting a gift in terms of the client's age, sex, race, ethnicity, religion, national origin, indigenous heritage, or sexual orientation?
- How well can you defend your acceptance or rejection of a gift to your professional peers? Think how you would feel if you read a story of yourself describing the gift that you accepted.
- What is in the client's best interest?

Special Requests

Clients occasionally make special requests for therapists to step outside traditional therapeutic settings. Such requests often involve upcoming special events in the client's life. Special events can be conceptualized on a continuum that includes formal public events or ceremonies (e.g., graduations, weddings, funerals) at one end of the continuum and private personal events (e.g., lunch, walk in the park) at the other end. Between these two extremes are informal events where other witnesses are present. In general, the greater the formality and publicity, the greater the likelihood there will be witnesses and the less likely that any interaction will be subject to misinterpretation by the client or others. Conversely, the more informal and private the event, the more likely the interaction will be highly personalized and subject to possible misinterpretation. Table 3 (below) illustrates four types of special events based on the dimensions of publicity (public vs. private) and formality (formal vs. informal).

Table 3: Types of Special Events

	Public	**Private**
Formal	Public formal	Private formal
Informal	Public informal	Private informal

Table 3 depicts four types of special events, each of which is illustrated by one of the following examples: A *formal public* event might include a ceremony such as a graduation, wedding, or funeral, whereas an *informal public* event might include an open house, dinner party, or an informal faith-based organizational activity. A *formal private* event might include a hospital visit or a home visit based on clinical necessity, whereas an *informal private* event might include having coffee or dinner with a client. This method of classifying special events is not meant to imply that any of the preceding types of events is ethical or unethical, but simply to clarify the differences between the types.

Pope et al.'s (1987) national survey of professional psychologists revealed that 20.4% of professional psychologists reported "going to a client's special event (e.g., wedding)" and 28.7% of the respondents agreed that "going to a client's special event (e.g., wedding)" was ethical "under many circumstances" (Pope et al., 1987). Using the classification scheme in Table 3, a wedding would be considered an example of a formal public event (i.e., a ceremony). Similarly, high school graduations, Bar/Bat Mitzvahs, and funerals would also be considered formal public events or ceremonies. The boundaries of public ceremonies are less likely to be subject to misinterpretation by the client or others. In contrast, a client's social party would be classified as an informal public event, in which the informality of the setting and less stringent boundaries could more easily lead to misinterpretation or other boundary crossings. Pope et al.'s (1987) survey revealed that 4.4% of professional psychologists reported "accepting a client's invitation to a party" and only 10.7% of the respondents agreed that "accepting a client's invitation to a party" was ethical "under many circumstances" (p. 996). A national survey of certified counselors indicated that 86% of the participants reported that "going to a client's special event (e.g., wedding)" was ethical, whereas only 34% of the participants reported that "accepting a client's invitation to a party" was ethical (Gibson & Pope, 1993, p. 332). Clearly, the dimensions of publicity and formality are two important determinants of the perceived ethicality of client special requests.

Baird (2001) provides some useful guidelines for therapists when a request is made by a client to step outside the traditional therapeutic framework. First, look for a more traditional means of addressing the needs of the client within the context of psychotherapy. Ask yourself how the client's request can be addressed within a traditional therapeutic framework. Ask yourself in what ways the client's request reflects a desire on the part of the client for the therapist to meet the client's needs which are unmet by important people in the client's life. Interpret, rather than gratify, the client's request whenever appropriate. Examine your own motives and needs that might be influencing your decision to step outside the boundaries. As always, consult with a colleague before considering stepping outside traditional boundaries. Consider how decisions to step outside traditional boundaries will be viewed by colleagues. Remember that any subsequent allegations of misconduct are only strengthened when considered within the context of known boundary crossings in other areas of the therapeutic relationship. It may be helpful to talk with the client about issues that can arise if the client comes to expect equivalent behaviors from you in the future. If you decide to respond to a client's special request by stepping outside traditional boundaries, talk with the client first about the implications of such nontraditional therapist behavior. If you decide to step outside traditional boundaries, explore with the client afterwards about the impact of such boundary crossings on the therapeutic relationship.

When considering how to respond to a client's special request or invitation to attend a client's special event, ask yourself these questions:

- Is there an institutional policy regarding accepting clients' special requests or invitations? If an institutional policy forbids accepting the request or invitation to a special event, then don't attend.
- What is the symbolic value of the client's special request? What is the clinical significance of the client making the request or extending the invitation to the event?
- Where does the event occur on the continuum between privacy and publicity? Attending private events may create an appearance of impropriety, whereas attending a public ceremony would be less controversial.
- Is accepting the special request or accepting an invitation consistent with your theoretical orientation? If not, then don't attend.
- If accepting the client's special request or invitation is consistent with your theoretical orientation, then is it part of your treatment plan with a particular client? If it is not part of your treatment plan, then don't attend.
- If accepting the client's special request or invitation is part of your treatment plan, then is there a way to accomplish the same treatment objective without accepting the request or invitation? If there is another way to accomplish the objective, then consider using other methods first.
- How well are you managing clear boundaries and maintaining therapeutic neutrality? When in the process of therapy is the client making the special request or extending the invitation? What are your motivations for accepting the special request or invitation? If you are already having trouble managing boundaries, then don't attend.
- How intact are the client's ego boundaries, reality testing abilities, psychological strengths, and levels of functioning? In other words, are there any clinical contraindications regarding accepting the

client's special request or accepting the invitation? Are there any indications that the client might feel exploited or otherwise misinterpret your acceptance or decline of the special request? If the client has weak ego boundaries or distorted perceptions of reality, then consider the likelihood that accepting the request could result in confusion, misinterpretations, or distortions on the part of the client. On the other hand, consider that declining the client's special request could also result in consequences.

- What is the prevailing practice within the local community? In general, the more that the practice of complying with the special request or accepting an invitation is considered an acceptable practice within a local community, the more likely it will be perceived as an appropriate arrangement.
- What are the multicultural implications of accepting or declining the client's request? In other words, what is the significance of accepting or declining the request in terms of the client's age, sex, race, ethnicity, religion, national origin, indigenous heritage, or sexual orientation?
- How well can you defend your accepting or declining the request to your professional peers? Think how you would feel if you read a story of yourself describing your compliance with a client's special request or attendance at a client's special event.
- What is in the client's best interest?

SUMMARY OF
MANAGING BOUNDARIES

Just as good fences make good neighbors, good boundaries make a firm foundation for a good relationship in psychotherapy. Although ethical practice requires boundary management, there may be times when boundaries are sometimes crossed for the purpose of serving the best interests of the client. Boundary crossings involve changes in a professional's role that can potentially benefit a client, whereas boundary violations involve unethical actions that harm or exploit clients. Boundary crossings are not necessarily unethical, but they may become problematic because they can sometimes lead to a slippery slope that results in a boundary violation, intentional or otherwise. Boundary violations are always unethical, because they always exploit the client at some level. One of the best ways to avoid boundary violations is to avoid boundary crossings. Dual or multiple role relationships occur when a professional assumes two or more roles at the same time or sequentially with a client or with someone who has a significant relationship with the client. Dual roles are not necessarily unethical, but they may become problematic. However, there are some prohibited dual roles that are always unethical because they may harm or exploit clients. One of the best ways to avoid prohibited dual relationships is to avoid dual relationships in the first place. When a dual relationship is unforeseeable, one of the best ways to avoid a problematic dual relationship is to manage the duality through consultation with an experienced colleague. Dual relationships can lead to conflicts of interest, and conflicts of interest can be avoided by doing a conflicts check when working with clients. One of the risk factors for boundary problems involves ethical blind spots, which can often be identified through supervision, peer consultations, and personal psychotherapy. When managing boundaries, always consider the best interests of the client.

POINTS TO REMEMBER

- Good boundaries make a firm foundation for a good relationship in psychotherapy.
- Boundary crossings involve changes in role that can potentially benefit a client.
- Boundary violations are unethical breaches that harm or exploit clients.
- The best way to avoid boundary violations is to avoid boundary crossings.
- Dual relationships are not necessarily unethical but they may become problematic.
- There are some prohibited dual relationships that are always unethical.
- Conflicts of interest can be avoided by doing a conflicts check when working with clients.
- Ethical blind spots can often be identified through peer consultations.
- Always consider the best interests of the client.

Chapter Four

Ethical Decision Making: Doing the Next Right Thing

"Always do right. This will gratify some people, and astonish the rest," advised Mark Twain (1901) in his message to the Young People's Society. Yet how does one always do right? Ethics is about so much more than doing right and avoiding bad behavior. It is about skillfully thinking through the shades of gray in a decision-making paradigm. Ethical decision making can be an interesting deductive process if one has the right conceptual tools. There are several basic conceptual tools for addressing the gray areas of complex ethical dilemmas. Although ethical standards are printed in black and white when they are published in the pages of an ethics code, it is usually the shades of gray between the lines that are encountered in everyday clinical practice.

Professionals striving for the highest standards of care may be interested in using an ethical problem-solving and decision-making approach to ethics. An underlying assumption regarding ethical decisions is that they are based on *principles*. Under ideal conditions, one should be able to specify the principles upon which an action is based. Two cornerstones of good ethical decision making include *knowledge* (knowledge competencies) of ethical standards and *proficiency* (skill competencies) in implementing a decision-making process. One's knowledge of standards should include an understanding of the difference between *mandatory* and *aspirational* ethical obligations. Aspirational obligations represent ethical ideals or the ethical "ceiling" of behavior, whereas mandatory requirements represent minimal standards or the "floor" of ethical behavior (Haas & Malouf, 2005). Aspirational ethical obligations represent the highest ideals of excellence embodied in the five general statements contained in the APA (2002) Ethical Principles, whereas *mandatory* requirements represent the enforceable ethical standards delineated in the more specific Ethical Standards and Code of Conduct. For purpose of clarity throughout this chapter, the term Ethical Standard is used to refer to any of the specific standards contained in the APA Code of Conduct. The term Ethical Principle is used to refer to any of the five General Principles, as well as what are often described as overarching moral principles (Haas & Malouf, 2005; Meara, Schimdt, & Day, 1996). Overarching moral principles refer to principles such as autonomy, beneficence, nonmaleficence, justice, fidelity, and veracity.

In learning to identify mandatory requirements, it may be helpful to consult the official ethical standards of one's profession. Because mandatory ethical standards are incorporated into statutory laws in many states, one should also be familiar with regulatory laws governing practice in one's state. Those interested in a more aspirational level of ethical awareness might be interested in reviewing literature such as *Ethics for Psychologists: A Commentary on the APA Ethics Code* (Canter et al., 1994), *Ethical Conflicts in Psychology* (Bersoff, 2003), and the *ACA Ethical Standards Casebook* (Herlihy & G. Corey, 2006), which contain practical case discussions, empirical research, and scholarly commentaries related to various ethics topics.

Although knowledge of professional codes of conduct and their overarching ethical principles provide guidelines for aspirational and mandatory behavior, relying only on ethical standards may be open to criticism because such standards define only the minimally acceptable level of actions. Furthermore, because there are many practical situations that are not clearly addressed by specific ethical standards, there is often a need for specific decision-making guidelines in the gray areas. As Herlihy and G. Corey (2006) point out, "When we find ourselves navigating in waters not clearly charted by our profession's *Code of Ethics*, we must be guided by an internal ethical compass" (p. 14). One such "internal ethical compass" may involve a set of decision-making rules by which ethical standards can be applied to practical situations.

The APA (2002) *Ethical Principles of Psychologists and Code of Conduct* are intended to provide general principles and specific standards to cover most situations encountered by psychologists. The Preamble offers the following guidelines:

> The development of a dynamic set of ethical standards for psychologists' work-related conduct requires a personal commitment and lifelong effort to act ethically; to encourage ethical behavior by students, supervisees, employees, and colleagues; and to consult with others concerning ethical problems. (p. 1062)

Although the APA Preamble contains some guidelines for "the development of a dynamic set of ethical standards," the Ethical Principles themselves do not contain a formal decision-making model. For this reason, other resources must be used to guide ethical decision making in the gray areas not addressed by specific standards. A review of the literature reveals several resources that practitioners consider to be useful in ethical decision making. In a national survey of professional psychologists (Pope et al., 1987), respondents indicated that informal networks of colleagues are often viewed by psychologists as the most effective form of guidance. Listed in descending order from the most to the least effective sources of information for making ethical decisions, respondents in the survey reported that they relied on formal APA Ethical Standards, internships, APA Ethics Committee, graduate programs, agencies, state ethics committees, continuing education programs, published clinical and theoretical work, and other less effective sources. Given that psychology is identified as an empirically based profession, it is interesting to note that published research was rated as less effective than other sources of information. As Pope et al. point out, "It is possible that research too rarely addressed ethical concerns and standards of practice in a way that is useful to psychologists" (1987, p. 1004). For certified counselors, the most valued resources relied on for making ethical decisions are reported to be formal ethical standards of the profession, the national ethics committee, the *Journal of Counseling and Development*, state licensing boards, and colleagues (Gibson & Pope, 1993).

PRINCIPLE ETHICS
AND VIRTUE ETHICS

In the study of ethics, there is a distinction made between principle ethics and virtue ethics. *Principle ethics* involves the study of ethical principles and professional standards, whereas *virtue ethics* refers to the development of character virtues and a sense of ethical self-awareness. Principle ethics, which include knowledge of applicable laws and ethical standards, are mainly the focus of this book. Virtue ethics, which are based more on character and a sense of ethical self-awareness, have received particular attention in the fields of organizational psychology, executive coaching, and psychotherapy. In the fields of business and politics, media attention has focused not so much on the presence of virtue but more on its absence. The absence of virtue has received considerable media attention in our nation's epidemic of corporate scandals. The term "business ethics" has almost become an oxymoron. It is not so much a matter that ethical standards have not existed so much as it is a matter that they have not been followed by many of our leaders.

Sternberg (2003) notes that some people (particularly executives and professionals) may be particularly susceptible to certain fallacies in thinking because, at least in some parts of our society, "they have been so rewarded for their intelligence that they lose sight of their humanity" (p. 5). In other words, they are so focused on their strengths that they are blind to their weaknesses. Professionals who are blind to their weaknesses will be overcome by them. Sternberg points out the dangers in the fallacies of thinking known as egocentrism, omniscience, and omnipotence. According to Sternberg, *egocentrism* involves taking into account one's own interests, but not taking into account the interests of others. The fallacy of *omniscience* involves the belief that one knows about everything, when in fact one may only know a lot about a little. The fallacy of *omnipotence* involves the grandiose belief that one is all-powerful and can do whatever one wants to do. These fallacies of thinking lead to arrogance, and arrogance leads to ethical slippage. Sternberg's research confirms the ancient wisdom: "Pride goeth before destruction, and an haughty spirit before a fall" (Proverbs 16:18).

How does one detect egocentrism, guard against arrogance, and learn to see one's ethical blind spots? When I asked this question to a respected colleague, my colleague advised me to strive for humility, surround myself with the wisdom of others, and listen to the counsel of others. In my consulting practice, I am often inspired by the character, common sense, and wisdom of my most respected colleagues. The true leaders of our field are the ones who inspire and encourage others by their actions. It is not simply the way ethical role models "talk the talk" but rather the way they "walk the walk" that provides us with wisdom and inspires us to do our best. To use a metaphor, principle ethics are based on knowledge that is in the head, whereas virtue ethics are based on character that is in the heart.

TELEOLOGICAL AND DEONTOLOGICAL ETHICS

In the study of philosophy, there are two types of moral justification, known as *teleological* justification and *deontological* justification. Teleological ethics (from the Greek *telos*, "end"; *logos*, "science") involves theories of morality that derive duty or moral obligation from what is good or desirable as an end to be achieved. It is the *consequences of actions* that determine their moral worth. From a historical perspective, teleological justification is based on the concepts of Jeremy Bentham's (1863/1948) universalistic hedonism ("The greatest happiness of the greatest number is the foundation of morals and legislation") or John Stuart Mill's (1863/2001) utilitarianism ("Act so as to achieve the greatest possible balance of pleasure over pain for all sentient creation"). Utilitarianism means promoting the greatest good for the greatest number of people. In other words, an action is ethical if it results in the creation of more good than harm. The teleological position is reflected in the statement "the ends justify the means."

Deontological ethics (from the Greek *deon*, "duty"; *logos*, "science") holds that the basic standards for an action's being morally right or wrong are independent of the good or evil consequences that are generated by the action. Deontology is based on duties, or actions or moral obligations that a person has toward another person, such as the duty to be honest. An action is ethical if it manifests one of a small set of primary moral characteristics. Etymologically, duties are actions that are due or owed to someone else, such as paying a debt of money that one owes to a creditor. In a broader sense, duties are simply actions that are morally mandatory. In other words, it is the moral basis of actions that determine their moral worth. From a historical perspective, deontological justification is based on concepts such as Immanuel Kant's (1785/2002) Categorical Imperative, as expressed in the Formula of the Law of Nature: "Act as if the maxim of your action were to become through your will a universal law of nature." Rather than the consequences of actions determining their moral worth, there is an emphasis on the moral basis of consequences. An action may be ethical regardless of its outcome.

Teleology and deontology are not just lofty abstract concepts; they are processes that operate in concrete ways in the real world. When a therapist decides whether or not to take an action (such as warning a readily identifiable third party of a client's specific threat of imminent and foreseeable violence) that may result in harm to his or her client (such as being the victim of the third party's preemptive violence inflicted on the client), then the therapist is concerned with making a teleological decision, which is based on consideration of possible consequences. When a therapist decides to take an action that is required (such as legally mandated reporting of a reasonable cause to believe that a child has been abused), then the therapist is making a deontological decision, which is based on the ethical duty or requirement regardless of consequences. In teleological decision making, the therapist is concerned about the consequences of actions. In deontological decision making, the therapist is concerned with the ethical duty or basis of actions.

Determining the ethicality of one's actions becomes difficult when more than one principle is involved. The problem with a purely teleological position is expressed in the question, "Who is entitled to judge the outcome of a moral choice?" On the other hand, the problem with a purely deontological position is that it provides no decision rules for selecting the most ethical action when each choice is based on a different moral ground. For this reason, ethical decision making must take into account both teleology and deontology. In reality, ethical actions are not based solely on either a deontological or a teleological position. Rather, ethical actions are based on consideration of ethical principles *and* their consequences. Ethical actions are based on consideration of overarching moral principles and ethical standards (deontological ethics) within the context of their anticipated consequences (teleological ethics). Combining both approaches at their most basic levels, ethical decision making involves two questions: (a) What are the standards or principles that apply to this particular situation? (b) What are the best ways of balancing the standards and principles to ensure the best consequences (doing good and avoiding harm) to the persons involved?

A review of the literature reveals several decision-making models, ranging from the simple to the complex. Several of these models will be briefly described below.

SOME BASIC
DECISION-MAKING MODELS

One-Step Model

The most basic ethical decision-making model is reflected by one of the most frequently asked questions at ethics seminars: "Is it ethical to [fill in the blank]?" This type of question reflects a level of ethical awareness that is only slightly above the minimal level suggested by the negative form of the question: "Is it unethical to [fill in the blank]?" This level of ethical thinking is so simplistic that the most appropriate response is often an equally simplistic, "Just say no." In other words, "Whatever you are thinking about doing, don't do it."

Ethics questions are sometimes asked in a manner that implies a dichotomous "yes or no" response. Particularly when working in the ambiguous world of psychotherapy, where there are often no clear right or wrong answers, clinicians often want more certainty when it comes to answering ethics questions. Clinicians often want black-and-white answers to complex ethical questions, but often there aren't any. In reality, answers to ethics questions are usually deeper, broader, and more complex than what on the surface appear to be simple questions. Ethical decisions are not based on a vertical dichotomy of "ethical versus unethical." Instead, ethical decisions are based on a horizontal continuum of "highly aspirational" on the upper end and "completely unethical" on the lower end, with many varying shades of gray in between the two extremes.

Two-Step Model

Kitchener's (1984) model provides an example of a relatively simple, two-step decision-making process related to moral judgments. Kitchener describes two levels of moral thinking: an immediate intuitive response and a critical-evaluative level of thinking. The *intuitive* level represents ordinary or perhaps immediate moral judgments that include the "shoulds" and "musts" of morality. The *critical-evaluative* level comprises three components: rules and codes, ethical principles, and ethical theory. When considering conflicting values, client rights, and therapist responsibilities in a particular situation, the ethically conscientious practitioner may modify or qualify his or her immediate intuitive response on the basis of critical-evaluative thinking, even though the initial response may be ethically acceptable.

As previously mentioned, another two-step approach involves the two basic questions that can be derived from the combined perspectives of deontology and teleology. With this framework, ethical decision making essentially involves two questions: (a) What are the standards or principles that apply to this particular situation? (b) What are the best ways of balancing the standards and principles to ensure the best consequences (doing good and avoiding harm) to the persons involved?

Three-Step Model

Pope and Vasquez (1998) suggest a relatively straightforward decision-making approach that focuses on one's feelings, cognitions, and actions in response to specific ethical dilemmas. In their chapter on multiple relationships, Pope and Vasquez provide several case scenarios, each of which is followed by a series of discussion questions. Although the discussion questions are more complex, a simple three-step approach to decision making can be derived from them. When facing an ethical dilemma, ask yourself at least these three questions: (a) "How do you *feel*?" (b) "What do you *think* you should do?" and (c) "What are your options for *actions*?" This three-step approach to solving ethical problems may appeal to cognitive-behavioral clinicians. It is also a useful model for generating discussion in ethics seminars and case conferences.

Another example of a three-step approach is Gottlieb's (1993) model, in which a decision-making process is applied to the specific topic of avoiding exploitive dual relationships. Gottlieb's model is based on three dimensions that are considered important when a therapist is considering entering a dual relationship. This approach may be useful to psychotherapists contemplating a posttherapeutic relationship, such as a social relationship after therapy has been terminated. Although the model was designed for therapists considering engaging in posttherapeutic dual relationships with former clients, the approach is also applicable to teachers considering postgraduation relationships with former students, such as a social relationship or employment, after a student has completed a training program. The first dimension involves the *power differential*, which refers to the difference in power that a psychotherapist has in relation to a client. The second dimension involves *duration of the relationship*, which is an aspect of power because it is assumed that power increases over time. The third dimension involves *clarity of termination*, or the likelihood that the therapist and client will have professional contact at some point in the future. The decision-making process involves considering the contemplated relationship as well as the current or recent professional relationship with respect to each of these dimensions.

Although Gottlieb's model involves three variables, the decision-making model involves four steps. The first step involves assessing the current relationship according to the three dimensions of power differential (low, mid-range, and high power), duration of relationship (brief, intermediate, long duration), and specificity of termination (specific, uncertain, and indefinite termination). From the perspective of the client, where does the relationship fall on each of these dimensions? The second step involves examining the contemplated relationship along the three dimensions, as was done for the current relationship. The third involves examining both relationships for role incompatibility, particularly if the professional relationship involves a high power differential, long duration of relationship, and indefinite termination of the therapeutic relationship. The final step involves obtaining consultation from a colleague and examination of both relationships for role incompatibility before proceeding with the contemplated relationship.

Four-Step Model

Doverspike (2004c, 2005b, 2006a) uses a four-step model when discussing options for addressing complex ethical dilemmas faced by colleagues. This model has been used in case discussions in collegial consultations, continuing education seminars, and graduate school ethics courses. Table 4 (below) depicts what has been described as the 2 x 2 Factorial Matrix, which lends itself to a visual illustration that can be used in training programs and ethics seminars. It consists of an analysis of the pros (benefits) and cons (risks) of a given course of action in a specific situation. It offers an operational way in which one can implement the consequential "projective retrospective" style of consequential thinking. The four-factor model is most useful when the clinician is faced with making choices between alternative actions in a specific situation. To a large extent, the model is based less on ethical principles and more on a consequential analysis of the risks and benefits of various courses of action. In other words, it offers a visual representation of a consequential or teleological analysis of behavior. Table 4 illustrates the 2 x 2 Factorial Matrix based on the dimensions of contemplated actions ("Just do it" vs. "Don't do it") and consideration of consequences (benefits vs. risks).

Table 4: The 2 x 2 Factorial Matrix

	Just Do It	**Don't Do It**
Benefits	Benefits of Action	Benefits of Inaction
Risks	Risks of Action	Risks of Inaction

Table 4 depicts one way of considering the benefits and risks of a given course of action in a specific situation. Each course of action can be illustrated by one of the following examples. Consider the scenario in which a therapist is faced with the dilemma of deciding whether to take an action such as warning a readily identifiable third party of a client's specific threat of imminent and foreseeable violence. Assume that the action being contemplated involves warning the intended victim or target person, which would be illustrated as "Just do it" in Table 4. The benefits of warning the intended victim might include protecting the intended victim and thereby protecting the client from committing an action that could eventually harm the client (e.g., retaliatory aggression, prison sentence, and so forth). On the other hand, the benefits of not warning the intended victim (i.e., "Don't do it") might include protecting the client's privacy interests, maintaining confidentiality, building trust in the therapeutic relationship, and possibly reducing the risk of a third party's preemptive violence inflicted on the client. The risks of warning the intended victim might include violating the client's privacy, breaching confidentiality, eroding trust in the therapeutic relationship, and possibly precipitating a third party's preemptive strike against the client. Conversely, the risks of not warning the intended victim might include allowing harm to befall the intended victim and thereby creating harm to the client. The 2 x 2 Factorial Matrix can be useful during the final stage of ethical decision making when one is considering the relative benefits and risks of a specific course of action.

Another example of a different type of four-step model is found in Van Hoose and Paradise's (1979) *Ethics in Counseling and Psychotherapy: Perspectives in Issues and Decision Making*. In describing the characteristics of the ethically responsible professional, Van Hoose and Paradise suggest that a counselor "is probably acting in an ethically responsible way concerning a client if (1) he or she has maintained personal and professional honesty, coupled with (2) the best interests of the client, (3) without malice or personal gain, and (4) can justify his or her actions as the best judgment of what should be done based upon the current state of the profession" (p. 58).

Multistep Models

In their commentary on the APA Ethics Code, Canter et al. (1994, pp. 3-7) describe a seven-step decision-making process that emphasizes knowledge of ethical standards, state and federal laws and regulations, and institutional rules and regulations. The seven steps are as follows:

1. Know the Ethics Code.
2. Know the applicable state laws and federal regulations.
3. Know the rules and regulations of the institution where you work.
4. Engage in continuing education in ethics.

5. Identify when there is a potential ethical problem.
6. Learn a method for analyzing ethical obligations in often complex situations.
7. Consult with professionals knowledgeable about ethics.

The process recommended by Canter et al. is not so much a formal decision-making model as it is a set of recommendations for promoting ethical practice. The authors devote little attention to the skills needed to resolve complex ethical dilemmas. Although Canter et al. acknowledge that there are "numerous systems for formal analysis and resolution of ethical problems and dilemmas" (p. 6), the authors conclude that a detailed discussion of such systems is beyond the scope of their book.

A review of the literature indicates the availability of a variety of formal decision-making models that share several common features (G. Corey et al., 2007; Doverspike, 1999b; Haas & Malouf, 2005; Hill et al., 1995; Keith-Spiegel & Koocher, 1985; Kitchener, 1984; Koocher & Keith-Spiegel, 1998; Remley & Herlihy, 2005; Sinclair et al., 1987; Tymchuk, 1986; Welfel, 2006; Younggren, 2002a). The common features of these models include a sequential decision-making process involving identification of the affected parties and ethical principles involved in the decision, consideration of alternatives, choice of appropriate actions, and evaluation of consequences. Ethical decisions may be made quickly in most situations although more time-consuming, careful deliberation may be required in more complex situations. Relatively quick decisions can usually be made in situations in which there are clear-cut standards that do not conflict with each other. More careful consideration may be required in more complex situations in which there are ethical principles that conflict with each other. In such situations, consultation with a colleague can increase one's objectivity in the ethical decision-making process.

The Canadian Psychological Association (CPA; 2000) *Code of Ethics for Psychologists* continues to be one of the few mental health professional codes that contains a formal, detailed decision-making model. Based on earlier models proposed by others (Sinclair et al., 1987; Tymchuk, 1986), the Canadian model outlines several steps that typify the ethical decision-making process. The following outline summarizes the ethical decision-making model based on the Canadian *Code of Ethics*, with each section representing one of the steps contained in the model. In providing some commentary and discussion of each of these steps, I have integrated ideas from decision-making models proposed by other writers (Canter et al., 1994; Haas & Malouf, 2005; Keith-Spiegel & Koocher, 1985; Kitchener, 1984; Koocher & Keith-Spiegel, 1998; Remley & Herlihy, 2005). I have also relied heavily on Haas and Malouf's (2005) text *Keeping Up the Good Work: A Practitioner's Guide to Mental Health Ethics.*

AN ETHICAL
DECISION-MAKING MODEL

Identify the Affected
Parties Involved

The first step in making a decision involves identifying the individuals or groups that need to be considered in order to arrive at a solution to the ethical dilemma (Sinclair et al., 1987). Haas and Malouf (2005, p. 9) use the term *stakeholders* to refer to those parties who have legitimate stakes in the outcomes of a situation. Although traditional stakeholders include the therapist and the client, legitimate stakeholders may also include significant others, those who are likely to be affected by the situation, and other parties who contract or pay for services. Like good treatment planning, good decision making involves consideration of the preferences of others, particularly in terms of rights and responsibilities involved. Koocher and Keith-Spiegel (1998) recommend that the clinician evaluate the rights, responsibilities, and welfare of all affected parties. Sinclair et al. recommend that clinicians "take each of these individuals/groups in turn and explain in detail what consideration each is owed and why" (1987, p. 6).

In my own consultations with colleagues, one of the first questions I ask is, "Who is the client?" There are some ethical dilemmas that can be resolved by simply clarifying who is the client and who is not the client. Similarly, there are many ethical dilemmas that can be *prevented* by simply clarifying *in advance* who is the client and who is not. For example, when bringing a collateral into a client's session, it is important to obtain informed consent of the collateral after clarifying the collateral's role. This informed consent process can be facilitated by the use of a document such as the APAIT Outpatient Services Agreement for Collaterals available at http://www.apait.org.

The question of who is the client must also be addressed from the perspective of multicultural diversity considerations, including "those based on age, gender, gender identity, race, ethnicity, culture, national origin, religion, sexual orientation, disability, language, and socioeconomic status" (APA, 2002, p. 1063). Notwithstanding the argument of Garcia et al. (2003, p. 270) that "no cultural variables are included in the analysis of a dilemma" using rational decision-making models, identifying the client requires an analysis of multiple factors including diversity considerations (e.g., age, race, ethnicity) as well as clinical considerations (e.g., diagnosis, ego strengths, boundary considerations).

Identify Ethically Relevant Principles

When confronting an ethical dilemma, refreshing one's memory by reviewing relevant standards can help improve one's ethical decision-making ability. Relatively quick decisions can usually be made in situations in which there are clear-cut guidelines or standards that do not conflict with each other. There are many occasions in which what initially appears to be an ethical problem turns out to be a procedural or technical problem. For example, choice of assessment instruments in a psychological test battery would usually be considered a technical decision rather than a decision involving an ethical standard. However, choosing to administer psychological tests to one but not both parents in a child custody evaluation would require an ethical decision-making process.

In my own consultations with colleagues, one of the first questions I ask is, "What is the ethical standard that applies to this situation?" When one is not even aware there *is* a standard, then knowing how to follow the standard is difficult if not impossible. If a single relevant standard applies in a particular situation, one's first question should be, "Is there a reason to deviate from the standard?" (Haas & Malouf, 2005, p. 12). If there is no single ethical principle that applies to the situation, one's next step would involve identifying the relevant ethical dimensions that make the issue problematic.

Consider Personal Biases, Stresses, and Self-Interest

When a practitioner is involved in making an ethical decision, the practitioner should always consider how his or her personal biases or self-interests might influence the development of courses of action or the choice among various courses of action. In other words, "Never let your sense of morals get in the way of doing what's right" (Isaac Asimov, attributed). In advising practitioners to consider their own personal biases and self-interests, the Canadian Psychological Association (2000) ethical decision-making model contains a step that is not contained in some of the other decision-making models. This step in the decision-making process goes to the heart of virtue ethics in addition to using one's head in considering principle ethics. As discussed previously, virtue ethics refer to the development of character virtues and a sense of ethical self-awareness. For example, egocentrism, which involves taking into account one's own interests but not taking into account the interests of others, is one of the fallacies of thinking that Sternberg (2003) has discussed as a contributor to unethical behavior.

According to the CPA model, personal values influence "the questions psychologists ask, how they ask those questions, what assumptions they make, their selection of methods, what they observe and what they fail to observe, and how they interpret their data" (p. 22). Particularly from a risk-management perspective, practitioners can never be totally free of self-interest. However, because one's personal values and self-interests can influence the decision-making process, practitioners must cultivate a sense of ethical self-awareness and concern for the interests of the client. The ethically self-aware practitioner is aware of how his or her background and personal values affect objectivity in the decision-making process.

Although ethical problem-solving models can facilitate the decision-making process, such models are not without their limitations. Because decision-making models are based on rationality, there is no way to eliminate the possibility of "self-serving rationalization" (Haas & Malouf, 2005, p. 18). As George Moore (1900) once observed, "The wrong way always seems the more reasonable." The best protection against self-serving rationalization includes consultations with an objective and impartial peer who can see one's *ethical blind spots.*

In the absence of peer consultation, there is a *visualization technique* that can be helpful in improving one's objectivity in making good decisions (Doverspike, 1997c, 1999c). Visualize your most respected colleague sitting in the consultation room with you and your client. While picturing your colleague in front of you, think to yourself, "What would he or she do? What would he or she say?" If you're *still* not sure, you should definitely consult with a peer.

The visualization technique described above is similar to the "clean, well-lit room" standard described in Haas and Malouf (2005, p. 17). That is, would you defend your contemplated actions to a group of your peers in public? Haas and Malouf point out that, "While some unethical decisions could pass this standard, no ethical decision should fail it" (p. 17). In contrast to the *public* visualization technique, another approach involves a *private* visualization technique. The private process is described (M. Sauls, personal communication, November 7, 2005) as the "dark parking lot" approach and it is suitable for professionals who hold themselves to the highest standards regardless of what their most respected peers would think. The dark parking lot approach to ethical decision making exemplifies the adage, "Ethics are what you do when no one is watching." This approach essentially asks the question, "How will I be able to live with myself?" For example, assume that you are leaving a large parking lot late one night and you happen to bump a parked vehicle as you are backing out of your parking spot, which was out of sight of any witnesses (or security cameras). How would you feel? What would you think? What would you do? Would you call someone? Would you leave a note? Would you leave the scene? Most importantly, how would you feel about your decision when no one is watching?

**Develop Alternative
Courses of Action**

Consider your various options at choice points. Because there is often more than one right solution to an ethical problem, think of solutions by thinking divergently as well as convergently. *Convergent* thinking refers to systematic thinking, including inductive and deductive reasoning, which brings together information on solving a problem by focusing on a single correct answer. *Divergent* thinking refers to thinking that moves away in diverging directions with many possibilities, including spontaneous flexibility and brainstorming, in order to involve a variety of factors that may lead to novel or creative ideas and solutions. In other words, in divergent thinking, there is no one "right" answer to a particular problem, but instead there may be many right answers. Divergent thinking is required when dealing with the many situations in clinical practice in which no single ethical dimension seems to outweigh the others. In such situations, a "solution-generating" or "brainstorming" approach can be helpful and a variety of actions may prove to be ethically appropriate (Haas & Malouf, 2005, p. 15). In generating possible courses of action, one should consider a variety of actions regardless of whether such actions initially appear to be ethically appropriate. Koocher and Keith-Spiegel (1998) advise that this process "should be conducted without focusing on whether each option is ethical or feasible and may even include alternatives that might otherwise be considered useless, too risky, too expensive, or inappropriate" (p. 14). Koocher and Keith-Spiegel further point out that occasionally "an option initially considered less attractive may be the best and most feasible choice after all" (p. 14).

When faced with ethical dilemmas, colleagues are usually concerned with which actions to take. Practitioners typically ask the question, "What should I *do*?" When providing ethics consultations for colleagues, I always ask the question, "Have you considered doing nothing?" In generating possible courses of action, one should always consider the option of taking *no action at all*. Based on a problem-solving approach to psychotherapy, there are some problems for which the best solution may involve taking no action at all. In legal decision making, one should always consider the option of "not doing anything" or simply deferring a decision because such an option can sometimes achieve the desired outcome (R. Nash, personal communication, April 26, 1993). Of course, there are many situations that call for decisive action, but it is rarely a bad idea to at least consider the option of taking no action at all.

When an appropriate course of action seems unclear, it may be because there are competing ethical principles that must be identified and prioritized in order to be reconciled. In such situations, consultation with a colleague can be helpful in identifying and prioritizing various conflicting principles and developing alternative courses of action. Consultation with a colleague can range from a formal, paid, independent consultation to a more informal phone call in which two colleagues discuss various courses of action with respect to possible risks and benefits (B. Alexander, personal communication, April 26, 1993).

Consider Possible
Risks and Benefits

The Canadian ethical decision-making model largely incorporates Tymchuk's (1986) approach in its consideration of the likely "short-term, ongoing, and long-term consequences" of each course of action on the individuals or groups involved or likely to be affected (p. 40). The most important step in Tymchuk's model involves determining which alternative to implement by looking at the short-term, ongoing, and long-term consequences, and considering the likely psychological, social, and economic costs with a risk-benefit analysis of each alternative. In addition to enumerating consequences of each alternative, Koocher and Keith-Spiegel (1998) suggest that the clinician "present any evidence that the various consequences or benefits resulting from each decision will actually occur" (p. 14).

In considering the possible risks and benefits of a course of action, Stadler (1986) suggests that one apply three simple tests to the selected course of action to ensure that it is appropriate. Incorporating Stadler's tests into their own decision-making model, Herlihy and G. Corey (2006) offer the following guidelines:

In applying the test of *justice*, assess your own sense of fairness by determining whether you would treat others the same in this situation. For the test of *publicity*, ask yourself whether you would want your behavior reported in the press. The test of *universality* asks you to assess whether you could recommend the same course of action to another counselor in the same situation. If you can answer in the affirmative to each of these three tests and are satisfied that you have selected an appropriate course of action, then you are ready to move on to implementation. (p. 16, italics added)

Universality is typically what distinguishes *ethical* action from *expedient* action (Haas & Malouf, 2005). Ethical actions are based on universal moral principles that transcend a specific situation. Historically, the idea of universality in moral law dates back at least as early as the writings of John Stuart Mill (1863/2001). For the contemporary psychotherapist, ethical actions are based on universal ethical principles that are designed to protect the welfare of the client, whereas expedient actions are based more on factors such as pragmatism and practicality. The concept of universality is expressed by the question, "Would I wish my action to become a universal law?" (Eyde & Quaintance, 1988, p. 149). Haas and Malouf (2005) ask a similar question, "Would I recommend this same course of action to every other person essentially similar to me who is operating in essentially the same circumstances?" (p. 16).

The concept of universality must also be balanced with the concept of *diversity*. Although legal and ethical standards are applied universally, particularly with respect to the overarching moral principle of justice, the application of ethical standards must also take into consideration multicultural diversity differences such as "age, gender, gender identity, race, ethnicity, culture, national origin, religion, sexual orientation, disability, language, and socioeconomic status" (APA, 2002, p. 1063).

In considering the possible risks and benefits of one's actions, it may be helpful to engage in *consequential* thinking or projective-retrospective thinking. In my own consultations with colleagues, I often encourage consequential thinking by using the 2 x 2 Factorial Matrix illustrated in Table 4 (p. 91). Similar to a cost-analysis approach, the Factorial Matrix approach encourages the practitioner to evaluate the short-term and long-term benefits and risks of two different courses of contemplated action (e.g., "Just do it," "Don't do it").

Choose a
Course of Action

After considering possible risks and benefits of various alternatives, the next step involves choosing an appropriate course of action. Sinclair et al. (1987) recommend that clinicians consider the questions, "What is the minimal circumstance you can conceive in this situation which would lead you to a different choice of action? What would that action be? Why?" (p. 6). In choosing a course of action, one should consider whether the chosen course of action presents any *new* ethical problems (Haas & Malouf, 2005). If one anticipates that the chosen course of action might present any new problems, then it may be necessary for the clinician to retrace his or her steps by reviewing applicable standards, considering other alternatives, and obtaining peer consultation.

When encountering a situation in which there is a conflict between ethical standards, Haas and Malouf (2005) recommend that clinicians consider *overarching* ethical principles such as autonomy, responsibility, universality, nonmaleficence, and beneficence. Overarching ethical principles are embodied in the General Principles of the APA (2002) Ethical Principles, which refer to rights and responsibilities such as autonomy, beneficence and nonmaleficence, fidelity and responsibility, integrity, justice, and respect for people's rights and dignity. Meara et al. (1996) identify six overarching moral principles, including autonomy, beneficence, nonmaleficence, justice, fidelity, and veracity, the first four of which are emphasized in the biomedical ethical model of Beauchamp and Childress (2001). In plain English, each principle is described below in terms that are relevant to psychotherapy.

- *Autonomy* refers to the right and promotion of self-determination as evidenced by the freedom of an individual to make his or her own decisions and choose his or her own direction.
- *Beneficence* refers to promoting good for others and contributing to the welfare of others.
- *Nonmaleficence* refers to avoiding doing harm to others and refraining from actions that risk hurting others.
- *Justice* refers to providing fairness and equal access to all people, regardless of age, sex, race, ethnicity, religion, national origin, or sexual orientation.
- *Fidelity* refers to keeping one's promises, honoring one's commitments, and being faithful to one's responsibilities of trust in a relationship.

- *Veracity* refers to being honest, truthful, and trustworthy. Trust is required to build a relationship, and honesty is required to build trust.

When providing consultations for colleagues, I often ask the question, "What does the *client* want?" Of course, this does not mean that the therapist simply does what the client wants, but rather that the therapist respects the client's autonomy and right of self-determination. Although ethical decisions are driven by principles rather than personalities, autonomy *is* an overarching ethical principle. In other words, the client generally has the right to self-determination. In most situations involving competent and reasonable adults, client autonomy is usually given considerable weight in the decision-making process. Based on the principle of client autonomy, there should be maximum involvement of the client at every stage of the decision-making process (Hill et al., 1995). Client involvement in a collaborative decision-making process usually increases the likelihood of a positive outcome. The exception to this general rule would be in life-threatening situations, where there is a conflict between autonomy and beneficence. In an emergency, beneficence is usually given greater weight than autonomy.

Consider Community Standards

In considering various courses of action, one should also consider what others are doing. In other words, one should consider the prevailing professional community standards. One way to consider community standards is through a review of the literature on ethics beliefs and ethical behavior of mental health professionals. There are several studies that have surveyed mental health professionals including psychiatrists, psychologists, and social workers (Borys & Pope, 1989), professional psychologists (Pope et al., 1987), certified counselors (Gibson & Pope, 1993), and Christian counselors (McMinn & Meek, 1996).

Pope and colleagues (1987) reported the results of a survey of 456 professional psychologists concerning what they actually think and do in the real world of providing psychological services in everyday practice. Pope et al. surveyed members of APA Division 29 (Division of Psychotherapy) who responded to an 83-item survey in which the respondents were asked to identify their ethical beliefs and their actual behaviors in a variety of situations. Pope et al.'s list included 82 different items, with one item being repeated to allow for a reliability check.

With regard to what might be described as some of the most unethical behaviors identified by the Pope et al. survey, the following items are identified by the percentage of respondents who rated the behavior as *unquestionably not ethical*: engaging in sexual contact with a client (96.1%), engaging in erotic activity with a client (95.0%), disrobing in the presence of a client (94.7%), discussing a client (by name) with friends (94.5%), signing for hours a supervisee has not earned (92.5%), doing therapy under the influence of alcohol (89.5%), borrowing money from a client (86.2%), getting paid to refer clients to someone (88.4%), selling goods to clients (71.1%), allowing a client to disrobe (86.2%), engaging in sex with a clinical supervisee (85.1%), going into business with a client (78.5%), unintentionally disclosing confidential data (75.2%), giving a gift worth at least $50 to a client (69.7%), and making a custody evaluation without seeing the child (64.0%).

Although the Pope et al. survey did not focus on aspirational ethical behaviors, the following items are identified by the percentage of respondents who rated the behavior as *unquestionably ethical*: offering or accepting a handshake from a client (71.9%), breaking confidentiality if client is homicidal (69.1%), addressing a client by his or her first name (65.1%), breaking confidentiality to report child abuse (64.9%), having a client address you by first name (63.6%), filing an ethics complaint against a colleague (57.9%), breaking confidentiality if client is suicidal (57.5%), charging for missed appointments (45.8%), not allowing clients access to raw test data (36.8%), using a computerized test interpretation service (34.9%), being sexually attracted to a client (33.3%), and utilizing involuntary hospitalization (31.8%). Given technological changes that have occurred since these data were collected 2 decades ago, some of these percentages would probably be considered outdated. For example, using a computerized test interpretation service is currently a much more common practice than it was 20 years ago. Given changes in the legal landscape, including changes brought about by HIPAA and various state licensing board rules that incorporate the APA 2002 Ethics Code, some of the above "unquestionably ethical" behaviors (e.g., not allowing clients access to raw test data) would now be considered unethical and in violation of APA Ethical Principles and HIPAA federal regulations. It is important to note that not two but three revisions of the APA (1990, 1992, 2002) Ethical Principles have occurred since the publication of the APA (1981) standards that were in use at the time the Pope et al. survey was conducted.

Borys and Pope (1989) conducted a national study using the same survey instrument during the same time period with respondents from three major mental health professions (570 psychiatrists, 905 psychologists, and 658 social workers). Using the Therapeutic Practices

Survey, which measures both "ethics" (beliefs regarding the ethicality of a behavior) and "practices" (self-reported frequency of a behavior), Borys and Pope reported that a majority of the respondents rated five behaviors as never ethical. These behaviors are identified by the percentage of respondents who rated the behavior as *never ethical:* sexual activity with a client before termination of therapy (98.3%), selling a product to a client (70.8%), sexual activity with a client after termination of therapy (68.4%), inviting clients to a personal party or social event (63.5%), and providing therapy to an employee (57.9%). With respect to ethicality ratings, there were only two items for which less than 10% of the respondents rated a behavior as *never ethical*: accepting an invitation to a client's special occasion (6.3%) and accepting a gift worth less than $10 (3.0%). With respect to actual practices, there were only two behaviors in which a majority of the respondents reported having engaged with at least one client: accepting a gift worth less than $10 (85.2%) and providing concurrent individual therapy to a client's significant other (61.2%).

Gibson and Pope (1993) reported results of a national survey similar to the Pope et al. (1987) survey but with a more diverse sample of mental health professionals. Gibson and Pope added five behaviors at the end of the original 83 and replaced the repeated item, resulting in a total of 88 items. Gibson and Pope collected data from 579 counselors certified by the National Board for Certified Counselors (NBCC) concerning their beliefs about the 88 different behaviors. The participants indicated their beliefs about whether each of the 88 behaviors was ethical and also the degree to which they were confident of their judgment about the behavior. However, a limitation of the study was that the participants were questioned only about the perceived ethicality of the behavior and confidence of their judgment, but they were not questioned about the frequency of occurrence of the behavior in their actual practices. As Gibson and Pope emphasize, "Beliefs are not necessarily indicative of behavior" (p. 335).

With respect to behaviors that certified counselors in the Gibson and Pope survey overwhelmingly endorsed as ethical, there were a total of 11 items that at least 90% of the participants judged to be ethical. One-fourth of these items involved breaching confidentiality in cases of actual or potential harm to the client or a third party. The following items are identified by the percentage of respondents who rated the behavior as *ethical*: offering or accepting a handshake from a client (99%), joining a partnership that makes clear your specialty (98%), addressing client by his or her first name (97%), breaking confidentiality to report child abuse (96%), filing an ethics complaint against a colleague (96%), breaking confidentiality if client is homicidal (95%), having a client address you by your first name (95%), breaking confidentiality if client is suicidal (95%), using self-disclosure as a counseling technique (92%), advertising accurately your counseling techniques (90%), and charging for missed appointments (85%). With regard to behaviors that certified counselors overwhelmingly endorsed as not ethical, the following items are identified by the percentage of respondents who indicated "no" in response to whether or not a behavior was *ethical*: engaging in sexual contact with a client (0%), engaging in erotic activity with a client (0%), discussing a name of a client to a class you are teaching (0%), discussing a client by name with friends (1%), signing for hours a supervisee has not earned (1%), doing counseling while under the influence of alcohol (1%), tape recording client without consent (1%), and allowing a client to disrobe (2%).

McMinn and Meek (1996) reported results of a similar survey of 498 members of the American Association of Christian Counselors (AACC). McMinn and Meek used the same 88 items that were used in the Gibson and Pope survey, except that McMinn and Meek retained Pope et al.'s (1987) repeated item (#66 and #82: "Being sexually attracted to a client") rather than using Gibson and Pope's (1993) replacement item for #66 ("Advertising accurately your counseling techniques"). Of the 498 AACC members who responded to the McMinn and Meek survey, 77 were also members of the Christian Association for Psychological Studies (CAPS). McMinn et al. (1997) reported a comparison of responses to the 88-item survey between the total sample and the CAPS members.

With respect to behaviors that Christian counselors in the McMinn et al. (1997) survey overwhelming endorsed as ethical, the following items are identified by the percentage of the total sample (AACC and CAPS) and CAPS respondents, respectively, who rated the behavior as *unquestionably not ethical*: engaging in sex with a clinical supervisee (96%, 96%), engaging in erotic activity with a client (96%, 95%), disrobing in the presence of a client (96%, 93%), engaging in sexual contact with a client (95%, 96%), doing therapy under the influence of alcohol (94%, 95%), disclosing the name of a client to a class you are teaching (94%, 93%), allowing a client to disrobe (93%, 93%), signing for hours a supervisee has not earned (94%, 69%), borrowing money from a client (93%, 93%), discussing a client (by name) with friends (92%, 95%), leading nude group therapy or "growth groups" (91%, 89%), being sexually involved with a former client (87%, 82%), engaging in sexual fantasy about a client (85%, 78%), using sexual surrogates with clients (84%, 88%), giving a gift worth at least $50 to a client (79%, 82%), unintentionally disclosing confidential data (77%, 81%), getting paid to refer clients to someone (77%, 78%), telling client: "I'm sexually attracted to you" (77%, 66%), going into business with a client (74%, 80%), making custody evaluation without seeing child (70%, 76%), lending money to a client (68%, 72%), giving gifts to those who refer client to you (65%, 63%), doing custody evaluation without seeing both parents (59%, 57%), selling goods to clients (56%, 55%), going into business with a former client (48%, 51%), and accepting a client's gift worth at least $50 (45%, 48%).

Although the McMinn et al. survey did not focus on aspirational ethical behaviors, the following items are identified by the percentage of the total sample (AACC and CAPS) and CAPS respondents, respectively, who rated the behavior as *unquestionably ethical*: offering or accepting a handshake from a client (76%, 76%), breaking confidentiality to report child abuse (76%, 76%), breaking confidentiality if client is suicidal (74%, 81%), breaking confidentiality if client is homicidal (73%, 76%), addressing client by his or her first name (68%, 66%), joining a partnership that makes clear your specialty (59%, 68%), having a client address you by your first name (55%, 58%), using a computerized test interpretation service (46%, 54%), filing an ethics complaint against a colleague (45%, 55%), and charging for missed appointments (27%, 41%).

Because ethical beliefs are not necessarily indicative of ethical behavior, it may be useful to review how the AACC and CAPS respondents reported various behaviors. Fewer than 10% reported engaging in some behaviors, as indicated by the following items that are identified by the percentage of the total sample (AACC and CAPS) and CAPS respondents, respectively, who reported *never* engaging in these behaviors: engaging in sex with a clinical supervisee (100%, 100%), engaging in erotic activity with a client (99%, 97%), disrobing in the presence of a client (100%, 100%), doing therapy under the influence of alcohol (99%, 99%), disclosing the name of a client to a class you are teaching (99%, 100%), leading nude group therapy or "growth groups" (99%, 100%), borrowing money from a client (99%, 99%), using sexual surrogates with clients (98%, 99%), allowing a client to disrobe (98%, 99%), becoming sexually involved with a former client (98%, 97%), signing for hours a supervisee has not earned (97%, 54%), getting paid to refer clients to someone (96%, 97%), going into business with a client (95%, 95%), accepting a client's decision to commit suicide (94%, 99%), telling client: "I'm sexually attracted to you" (94%, 86%), discussing a client (by name) with friends (93%, 97%), giving a gift worth at least $50 to a client (93%, 95%), using a lawsuit to collect fees from a client (90%, 89%), making custody evaluation without seeing child (92%, 94%), kissing a client (92%, 91%), not disclosing your fee structure to a client (90%, 86%), giving gifts to those who refer client to you (90%, 80%), and accepting a client's gift worth at least $50 (93%, 95%).

McMinn et al. also reported some of the common behaviors of AACC and CAPS respondents, including the following behaviors which were reported occurring at least occasionally (i.e., including responses of *sometimes*, *fairly often*, and *very often*) among 90% or more of the respondents: hugging a client, using self-disclosure as a therapy technique, breaking confidentiality to report child abuse, addressing a client by first name or having a client address the therapist by first name, accepting a gift worth less than $5 from a client, and offering or accepting a handshake from a client. These reported behavior patterns are very similar to the patterns previously reported from surveys of professional psychologists (Pope et al., 1987).

Although ethical practice is based on principles rather than personalities, understanding what other professionals believe and how they behave can help provide some guideposts for ethical behavior. Good ethics are not based on the behavior of colleagues, but good ethics are sometimes reflected in the behavior of our most ethical colleagues.

Implement a
Course of Action

Although choosing a course of action is based on *principles*, implementing a course of action is often based on *pragmatism*. Implementation of a chosen course of action involves both practicality and prudence. *Practicality* refers to the likelihood that one can actually implement the course of action, whereas *prudence* refers to the fact that ethical decisions may at times be costly to the clinician who implements them (Haas & Malouf, 2005). Because ethical actions are based on the concept of universality rather than *expediency*, there are many situations in which an ethical course of action can be time-consuming, demanding, and costly. For example, asserting privilege and protecting confidential information in response to a subpoena can be emotionally demanding, time-consuming, and expensive for the clinician (Buchanan, 1997; DeFilippis et al., 1997).

In my own consultations with colleagues, I sometimes use role-playing to practice and sharpen the skills needed to implement a course of action. Implementing a course of action requires proficiency (skill competence) as well as understanding (knowledge competence). Implementation of an appropriate course of action typically requires "other (nonethical) skills such as assertiveness, tenacity, the existence of a supportive social network, and the ability to communicate one's chosen action in noncondescending and humane terms" (Haas & Malouf, 2005, p. 17).

Evaluate the
Results of Actions

Most ethical decision-making models conclude with an evaluation of the action taken. If one has engaged in *consequential* thinking prior to choosing a course of action, then it may be possible for one's actions to have fairly predictable results. However, good decisions can sometimes lead to bad results. One's best efforts can sometimes result in unintended or even adverse consequences. Evaluating the results of one's actions can lead to modification and improvement of the action plan.

In an article on preventing malpractice, Barnett (1997) concludes, "While psychologists are not required to guarantee positive outcomes, we must make a good faith effort to do so" (p. 22). In an ideal world, a clinician is held accountable not for the *accuracy* of his or her predictions but in the *reasonableness* that has been taken in arriving at such predictions. Reasonableness of behavior is of utmost importance in making ethical decisions (Behnke, 2004). Ethically responsible behavior is based on the assumption of a reasonable *effort*.

Assume Responsibility
For Consequences of Actions

Although the last step in most ethical decision-making models involves an evaluation of the action taken in a situation, the Canadian model addresses an important omission of other models. The last step in the decision-making process involves assuming responsibility for the consequences of one's chosen course of action. Assuming responsibility for one's actions may include correcting negative consequences, if any, which may have occurred as the result of one's actions (CPA, 2000). Alternatively, assuming responsibility may also involve continuing the decision-making process if the ethical issue itself has not been resolved satisfactorily. Finally, as Haas and Malouf (2005) point out, "It is also ethically incumbent on the responsible practitioner to learn from his or her mistakes" (p. 18). As a wise colleague once disclosed to me, "Good judgment comes from making mistakes. Great judgment comes from making big mistakes." My colleague's advice echoes the old adage, "Good judgment comes from experience; experience comes from bad judgment."

IDENTIFYING CONFLICTS
BETWEEN ETHICAL AND
LEGAL GUIDELINES

In their discussion of the limitations of ethical decision-making models, Haas and Malouf (2005) raise the question of whether a clinician can make a decision purely on the basis of ethical considerations without regard to legal standards. Their answer is an emphatic *no*. The authors recommend that the clinician first consider the purely ethical or moral aspects of the situation and then consider existing legal standards in terms of the implementation of the decision. On the other hand, Herlihy and G. Corey (2006) recommend that if a legal question exists, legal advice should be obtained first. Because mandatory ethical standards are incorporated into statutory laws in many states, a statutory code or legal reference book may be helpful. *The Psychologist's Legal Handbook* (Stromberg et al., 1988) is a good general resource regardless of the state in which one practices, and the APA Law and Mental Health Series of reference books are available for a total of 26 states. In Georgia, a desk reference such as *Law & Mental Health Professionals: Georgia* (Remar & Hubert, 1996) may be helpful in identifying applicable legal standards. In Florida, *Law & Mental Health Professionals: Florida* (Petrila & Otto, 2003) may be useful.

In their guidelines for ethical practice, Herlihy and G. Corey (1996) offer the following four steps for addressing decisions in which there are apparent conflicts among legal, ethical, and institutional forces:

1. *Identify the force that is at issue regarding the counselor's behavior.* Is the principle involved legal, ethical, employer imposed, or demanded by some other force?
2. *If a legal question exists, legal advice should be obtained.* If employed in an agency or institution, counselors should request legal guidance from their immediate supervisor. If in private practice, an attorney should be consulted.
3. *If there is a problem in applying an ethical standard to a particular situation or in understanding the requirements of an ethical standard, the best action a counselor could take is to consult* with colleagues and with those perceived to be experts in the counseling field. Once advice is sought and there seems to be a consensus on the appropriate response in an ethical dilemma, it is essential that the counselor take the advice given (Woody, 1988).

4. *If a force other than law or ethics* (for example, an employer, an accrediting body, or a funding agency) *is suggesting that a counselor take some action he or she perceives to be illegal, the counselor should seek legal advice* to determine whether such action is indeed illegal. If the action seems to be unethical, advice should be sought from colleagues or experts. In the event the counselor determines that an action is illegal or unethical, the counselor should approach the representative of the force in an attempt to resolve the problem in a satisfactory manner. If such an approach is unsuccessful, the counselor should seek legal advice regarding the next course of action. (pp. 288-289)*

PSYCHOLOGY AND
THE LAW

One of my respected colleagues once observed that psychologists are on the verge of practicing law when they provide peer consultations regarding legal questions such as mandated reporting of suspected abuse of minors, elders, and the disabled. I share my colleague's concern that many psychologists who request ethics consultations are in reality needing legal consultations. In my own experience, the majority of therapists who call to ask a "quick question" usually have a more complex legal question that is the crux of the matter. In fact, when conducting ethics workshops over the past several years, I try to avoid the "quick question" of the hallway consultation because in reality it is often the tip of the iceberg, under which lurks a more complex legal question complicated by clinical dynamics that would baffle even a master psychotherapist. Asking a psychologist for free legal advice is probably worse than asking an attorney for free psychotherapy.

In order to become licensed, psychologists are required to demonstrate *knowledge* of applicable statutory and case law (knowledge competency) as well as *proficiency* in being able to integrate and apply such knowledge in practice (skill competencies). For example, Georgia psychologists are required to pass the Georgia Jurisprudence Examination (see Paragraph 2[c] of Chapter 510-2-.01, Application by Examination), covering "current laws, rules and regulations, and general provisions." The APA (2002)

---

* From *American Counseling Association Ethical Standards Casebook* (5th ed., pp. 288-289), by B. Herlihy and G. Corey, 1996, Alexandria, VA: American Counseling Association (ACA). Copyright © 1996 by American Counseling Association. Reprinted with permission. No further reproduction authorized without written permission of the ACA.

Ethics Code explicitly states, "In the process of making decisions regarding their professional behavior, psychologists must consider this Ethics Code *in addition to applicable laws* [italics added] and psychology board regulations (p. 1062). An underlying assumption in the APA code is that psychologists *understand* applicable laws and legal regulations. In fact, the word "law" is explicitly stated approximately 30 times throughout the APA Ethics Code, which itself is incorporated into psychology board rules and regulations in approximately 27 states.

To know one's ethical duty, a practitioner must also understand his or her legal duty (Behnke, 2005). A good place to start is by learning the laws and knowing how to integrate them into one's practice. In other words, know the code. Keep a desk reference and then do your homework. Know which questions to ask when seeking a legal consultation—from an attorney. Get to know an attorney who has specialized knowledge and proficiency in mental health law. If you don't wish to retain a private attorney, then call the risk-management service provided by your professional liability insurance company. In either event, because there are significant differences in the statutory laws and legal precedents (case law) in different states, be sure to get a legal opinion based on the specific laws of the state in which you are practicing. Finally, remember that the most effective and least expensive form of liability insurance is good documentation (Schaffer, 1997). In plain English, keep good notes of your consultations, decisions, and actions. In my opinion, practitioners are not on the verge of practicing law when they discuss legal questions, but they are certainly on the verge of malpractice when they fail to provide a reasonable standard of care to their clients.

SOLVING ETHICAL PROBLEMS
BEFORE THEY ARISE

Although ethical decision-making models offer a *reactive* approach to ethical problem solving, clinicians should consider adopting a *proactive* approach to ethical decision making. Such an approach focuses on primary prevention of ethical problems by anticipating and handling potential ethical problems as procedural issues that are discussed and handled in advance. A working knowledge of relevant ethical and legal standards allows one to anticipate potential problematic situations before they arise. *Primary prevention* involves participating in ongoing continuing education, developing character virtue, and striving for excellence in practice. Examples of primary prevention might include attending ethics workshops, learning about new laws that govern practice, and managing client expectations in advance through the use of an adequate process of informed consent. *Secondary prevention* involves resolving ethical dilemmas and managing ethical problems as they arise in everyday practice. An example of secondary prevention might include consulting with an experienced colleague when faced with an ethical dilemma such as encountering an unforeseen dual relationship. *Tertiary prevention* involves intervention or learning from one's mistakes so they are not repeated in the future. An example of tertiary prevention might involve having to defend an ethics complaint and then later receiving an educative letter that provides some guidance in an area of deficiency of which the practitioner was not aware. It is sometimes said that good judgment comes from experience, and experience comes from bad judgment. When it is said that "Prevention is better than intervention" (C. Webb, personal communication, June 4, 2004), it means that primary and secondary prevention are better than tertiary prevention (i.e., intervention).

Although ethical decision-making models offer a reactive approach to ethical problem solving, clinicians should also consider using primary prevention to address ethical issues before they become problems. Most potential ethical problems can often be minimized or avoided altogether by discussing concerns at the outset. For example, potential misunderstandings related to fee disputes or financial arrangements can be addressed through the use of posted fee schedules and written financial agreements discussed prior to providing services. Potential misunderstandings related to limits of confidentiality can be addressed through the use of ongoing informed consent procedures. Anticipated problems related to issues such as limits of services or premature termination in managed care practice can be addressed in a collaborative manner at the outset of treatment. Potential problems related to dual relationships or boundary crossings can be avoided by adopting professional behavior and office policies that demonstrate clear limits and firm boundaries from the first session onward. As a general rule, most potential ethical problems can be avoided through the use of common sense, respectful attitudes, open communication, and ongoing consultation with colleagues.

SUMMARY OF
DECISION-MAKING GUIDELINES

In summary, ethical decision-making models can provide a framework for putting ethical principles into practice. Such models can be particularly useful in situations in which there are either conflicting standards or no clear standards at all. The common features of these models include a sequential decision-making process involving consideration of alternatives, choice of appropriate actions, and evaluation of consequences. When used appropriately, decision-making models can provide some helpful guidelines for achieving an aspirational level of ethical awareness. Although ethical decision-making models offer a reactive approach to ethical problem solving, clinicians should also consider adopting a proactive approach by using procedures that prevent ethical problems before they arise.

POINTS TO REMEMBER

- Identify the "stakeholders" or parties likely to be affected by the outcome of the situation.
- Identify relevant ethical principles and legal standards of practice.
- Use a "solution-generating" or "brainstorming" process to develop alternative courses of action.
- Consider short-term and long-term risks and benefits of each course of action.
- Choose an appropriate course of action in collaboration with the client.
- Implement the course of action with consideration to practicality and prudence.
- Conduct ongoing evaluation of the results of actions that can lead to modification or improvement of the action plan.
- Assume responsibility for consequences of actions. Learn from mistakes.
- Take a proactive approach in preventing ethical problems before they arise.

Chapter Five

Consulting With Colleagues: Don't Worry Alone

From time to time, everyone faces situations that require special consideration beyond one's own best judgment. The smart counselor learns from his or her mistakes; the wise counselor learns from the mistakes of others. The wise counselor also knows when to identify those situations that deserve consultation with a peer. Peer consultations are particularly important when clinicians must consider actions in high-risk situations (e.g., dispensing with informed consent, breaching confidentiality in a duty-to-protect situation, performing child custody evaluations, terminating with a noncompliant client). Two heads are usually better than one, and a brief consultation is better than none.

Peer consultation means talking with a respected colleague who is knowledgeable, objective, and impartial. It does not mean talking to someone who will simply agree with whatever actions you have already taken. Every practitioner faces complex situations that require consideration beyond one's own best judgment. The wise practitioner knows when to consult with a peer. A good peer is someone who can help you see a different perspective, identify your ethical blind spots, and maximize your options for responding to the situation. If you are not sure whom to call, one option is to call your state professional association's ethics committee and request an ethics consultation. As a confidential service to its members, most state professional associations' ethics committees have an ethics committee whose purpose is to provide ethics education and consultation to its members.

State professional associations' ethics committees have increasingly moved away from investigative and disciplinary roles toward more educative and consultative roles. There are several reasons for this trend. First, ethics committee members typically view themselves as educators and consultants rather than investigators or prosecutors. State professional association ethics committees usually view their primary role as promoting standards of the profession and encouraging their members to practice these standards, whereas state licensing boards usually view their primary role as protecting the public by enforcing professional standards and disciplining those who violate such standards. Similarly, the members of professional association ethics committees are volunteers whose primary interests are their members, whereas state licensing board members are political appointees whose primary oaths are sworn to the state government. In addition, because professional associations are composed of volunteers who work for intangibles, providing peer consultations is more rewarding and less time-consuming than conducting investigations into ethics complaints. Finally, many professional associations encourage educative peer consultations because such consultations are believed to reduce ethics complaints in the future. These reasons are consistent with the Preamble of the APA Ethics Code, which in part states, "The development of a dynamic set of ethical standards for psychologists' work-related conduct requires a personal commitment and lifelong effort to act ethically; to encourage ethical behavior by students, supervisees, employees, and colleagues; and to *consult with others concerning ethical problems* [italics added]" (APA, 2002, p. 1062).

Professional ethics committees usually perform two separate but related functions, including an adjudicatory role and an advisory role. The *adjudicatory* role, which in some respects is similar to one of the roles performed by state licensing boards, involves investigating and adjudicating ethics complaints against its members and, where appropriate, sanctioning members who are found to violate professional standards. The *advisory* role, which is very different from the primary role of a state licensing board, involves approving continuing education, ethics consultations, and advisory opinions to members of the organization. It is the advisory role that is relevant to the matter of consulting with colleagues. While providing collegial consultations or serving in an advisory role, members of professional ethics committees typically do not serve in investigative roles on the committee. Committee members who provide consultations, sometimes known as advisory opinions, are usually available to respond orally to inquiries on ethical issues from interested members of the professional organization. The name of the member requesting a collegial consultation or informal advisory opinion is usually held confidential unless the member elects otherwise. Ethics inquiries address prospective (not retrospective) conduct only. In other words, ethics consultations focus on contemplated courses of future actions rather than on retrospective analysis of past actions. The process is designed to assist practitioners in resolving ethical dilemmas before they rise to the level of ethical problems. If such matters do rise to the level of ethical problems, then the consultative process is designed to assist the practitioner in resolving the ethical problem before it rises to the level of an ethics complaint.

As explained in one state ethics committee's *Rules and Procedures*, "An informal oral opinion is the personal opinion of the responding Committee member and is neither a defense to a complaint nor binding on the full Ethics Committee (Georgia Psychological Association [GPA], 1996, p. 9). However, if a complaint should later be made against the member, the fact that the member made an informal inquiry and acted in accord with the informal opinion is considered by the Ethics Committee. As stated in the ethics committee rules, "The fact that a member relied on an informal advisory shall be given substantial weight by the full Committee in the event a complaint should later be made against the member for such conduct" (GPA, 1996, p. 10).

COMMON ETHICAL DICHOTOMIES

Ethical decision making is as much about asking the right questions as it is about finding the right answers. There is usually more than one solution to a problem, and the best way to discover the answers is to consult with a colleague. Consultation with a colleague may be helpful at any of the following steps in the decision-making process: (a) identification of relevant ethical or clinical standards (e.g., assessment of risk of violence vs. duty to protect third parties from imminent and foreseeable danger), (b) differentiation between ethical and legal issues (e.g., confidential communications vs. privileged information), (c) clarification of role expectations (e.g., primary client vs. collaterals), (d) clarification of conflicts of interest (e.g., multiple clients in a couple, marriage, or family), (e) identification of ethical blind spots, (f) identification of various courses of action ("brainstorming"), and (g) consideration of risks and benefits of action ("consequential thinking").

In my own consultations with colleagues, I have often observed some differences in the way that experienced colleagues obtain consultations compared to the way less experienced colleagues obtain consultations.

Less experienced colleagues seek consultations at the earlier steps of the decision-making process (e.g., identifying the relevant ethical standard, or differentiating between ethical and legal issues), whereas more experienced colleagues seem to seek consultations at the later steps of the decision-making process (e.g., identification of ethical blind spots, identification of courses of action, or consideration of benefits and risks). Compared to less experienced colleagues, their more experienced counterparts seem to seek consultation only after they have engaged in some careful consideration of a problem. In contrast, less experienced colleagues often seem to consult when they are getting started in the process (e.g., by relying on a more experienced consultant to identify the specific ethical standard or salient ethical dimension of a dilemma). It is often as if more experienced colleagues obtain consultations when they are putting the "finishing touches" on a complex decision, rather than using the consultation to get the decision-making process started in the first place. More experienced colleagues also seem to be able to tolerate ambiguity better than less experienced colleagues, who often seem to become frustrated by the lack of a simple definitive answer in response to a complex problem.

When providing ethics consultations, I have also noticed that many consultations seem to revolve around some basic dilemmas, which do not necessarily involve specific ethical standards but rather more general ethical principles related to values. Ethical principles do not exist within a vacuum, but rather the matter of values permeates the decision-making process. The following list includes five common dilemmas that are often encountered during ethics consultations with colleagues.

Ethics Versus Easy

Ethical actions are often more difficult to take than unethical actions, although easy actions can often lead to quick solutions. However, although ethical actions are often more difficult in the short term, they are often easier in the long term. For example, a counselor may receive a phone call from a client requesting that a portion of the client's record be faxed to the client's insurance company in order to expedite timely payment of a claim. It would be easy for the counselor to comply with the client's verbal request. However, most prevailing ethical standards require that the counselor obtain a written authorization for the release of confidential information. When making an ethical decision, put ethics before easy.

Ethics Versus Economics

Ethical decisions have economic consequences, and economic decisions have ethical consequences. Ethical actions often have short-term costs and long-term benefits, whereas economic actions often have short-term benefits at the expense of long-term gains. For example, a family therapist who declines to provide a forensic expert witness opinion on matters related to child custody or parental fitness may experience an immediate economic cost related to forgoing a lucrative expert witness fee. On the other hand, a family therapist who accepts the lucrative fee for such testimony may experience an immediate economic gain but may later experience a long-term economic loss when one of the litigants files a licensing board complaint related to the unethical blurring of therapeutic and forensic roles. When making an ethical decision, put ethics before economics.

Ethics Versus Expediency

Ethical actions are sometimes more complicated than unethical actions. Expedient actions often get the job done, but the actions are not always ethical. Ethical actions are based on principles, which are designed to protect the welfare of the client. Expedient actions are based more on factors such as pragmatics and practicality, which are designed to get the job done. For example, a pediatric neuropsychologist employed by a hospital may be asked by the hospital administrator to allow an unqualified student intern to serve as psychometrist because it will allow the hospital to provide screenings for more children in the hospital before a qualified psychometrist can be hired. In deciding how to respond to the request, the neuropsychologist should be guided by the ethical principles of maintaining integrity and promoting competence. When making an ethical decision, put ethics before expediency.

Ethics Versus Extraversion

Sometimes a charming, seductive, manipulative, or provocative personality can exert influence over a counselor's judgment. Ethical actions are based on principles, which are designed to be objective and universal. Practitioners have a duty to place ethical principles before charming personalities. Rather than being charmed by the personalities involved in the situation, consider the ethical principles that govern a situation. For example, a therapist who receives an invitation to attend the wedding, graduation, or awards ceremony of a client may feel the pull of the client's very charming personality, logical intellect, or high socioeconomic status. In deciding how to respond to the request, the therapist should be guided by the ethical principle of considering whether the contemplated boundary crossing will have any potential for harm, such as loss of objectivity or loss of effectiveness in ongoing psychotherapy with the client. To use an old adage, put principles above personalities. In making an ethical decision, put ethics before extraversion.

Ethics Versus Entertainment

Journalists and reporters usually want their stories to be more sensational, by revealing graphic details or patient identity. Ethical actions are based on protecting the welfare of the client, including protecting the client's privacy. Professional psychotherapists have a duty to place patient privacy above journalistic interests of sensationalism. For example, a highly competent psychologist with many published books may receive a television journalist's request to demonstrate a specialized technique on a nationally syndicated television show using one of the therapist's actual clients. In deciding how to respond to the request, the psychologist should be guided by the ethical principles of protecting privacy and avoiding harm to the client. When making an ethical decision, put ethics before entertainment.

TOP 10 REASONS
NOT TO CONSULT A COLLEAGUE

At an ethics workshop conducted collaboratively by members of a state professional association ethics committee and licensing board (L. Campbell et al., 1999), ethics committee member Tom McIntyre presented a list of the Top 10 reasons not to obtain a consultation with a colleague.* With his permission, the following represents a modification of Tom's Top 10 list with some explanatory comments of my own:

   1. *"When in doubt, it's easier to do nothing."* In ethical decision making, there are some situations in which the best course of action turns out to have been no decision at all. However, good de-

---

* Reprinted with permission.

cision making requires looking at *all* available options—including consulting with a colleague. Sometimes, consulting with a colleague *can* result in a decision to do nothing about a specific situation, but "doing nothing" on the advice of a colleague is better than doing nothing at all.

2. ***"I'm waiting for the ethics committee to call me."*** This reason is perhaps a holdover from the prosecutorial mentality of the days of the past when a state professional association's ethics committee's prime directive was an implicit "Don't call us; we'll call you." In recent years, most committees operate with a more proactive, educative, and consultative interaction between colleagues. Members of professional ethics committees prefer to hear consultation calls from interested practitioners rather than complaint calls from angry clients.

3. ***"I'm wanting to turn a boring ethical dilemma into an exciting malpractice suit."*** In other words, "When I get bored I like to stir up some excitement." If you like excitement, try hang-gliding. If you prefer a little boredom, consult with a colleague.

4. ***"I like to live dangerously."*** A variation on the theme of the excitement of malpractice, this reason applies to those of us who like to live on the edge. Colleagues giving this reason might also be expected to endorse test items such as "At times I have a strong urge to live dangerously and do something exciting." Even skydivers consult with each other when packing their chutes.

5. ***"Asking for advice ruins the spontaneity of my practice."*** Like good treatment planning, good ethical practice requires planning. Most ethical decision-making models encourage a "solution-generating" or "brainstorming" phase (Haas & Malouf, 2005, p. 15), in which a variety of actions should be considered regardless of whether such actions initially appear to be appropriate. Rather than stifling spontaneity, a good peer consultation actually *increases* creative thinking.

6. ***"I'm a doctor (i.e., I don't ask for advice)."*** Remember Kingsbury's (1987) *American Psychologist* article on the cognitive differences between psychologists and psychiatrists? Clinical psychologist and psychiatrist Steven Kingsbury made the distinction that physicians view science as a set of facts and a body of knowledge, whereas psychologists view science as a process and a method of inquiry. Sometimes it is helpful to think of an ethical consultation not as a search for the "right answer" but as a process of discovering various options. Sometimes there are *several* right answers.

7. *"I'm a flawless PhD (i.e., Psychologically High Deity)."* This is a variation on the preceding deity theme, which may correlate with the MMPI-2 item, "I am entirely self-confident." Remember the first *DSM-IV* (American Psychiatric Association, 2000, p. 717) criteria for Narcissistic Personality Disorder? A grandiose sense of self-importance can increase a clinician's potential for ethical violations. These observations are consistent with Sternberg's (2003) research related to the self-destructive consequences of egocentric thinking that takes into account one's own interests but does not take into account the interests of others. In other words, arrogance is an enemy of ethics.

8. *"My schedule book runneth over."* It may be instructive to remember the words of St. Francis de Sales (1567-1622), the 16th-century Bishop of Geneva, who once said, "Half an hour's meditation is essential except when you are very busy. Then a full hour is needed." In other words, a quick consultation may be more important when you are very busy than when you are not.

9. *"I don't have time."* In other words, why put off until tomorrow something that doesn't need to be done anyway? Besides, if anything is worth doing, it would have already been done.

10. *"It costs too much."* When someone doesn't want to do something, a bad excuse is as good as a good one.

TOP 10 REASONS
TO CONSULT A COLLEAGUE

Perhaps the most important reason to consult with a colleague involves the word *reasonable* itself. In the APA (2002) Ethics Code, the words "reasonable" and "reasonably" appear approximately 28 and 13 times, respectively. Similarly, the words "appropriate" and "appropriately" occur 47 and 5 times, respectively. In the ACA (2005) Code of Ethics, the words "reasonable" and "reasonably" appear approximately 24 and 7 times, respectively, and the words "appropriate" and "appropriately" occur 73 and 4 times, respectively. In other words, for counseling psychologists who may be members of both organizations, there would be over 200 reasons to obtain ethics consultations, and this estimate does not even include the more numerous clinical and technical reasons for obtaining consultations. A good rule of thumb is "Consult a colleague whenever the word *reasonable* appears." The word "reasonable" does not define itself, but is often defined in a circular manner as "what a reasonable person would do." Because what is reasonable to one may not be reasonable to another, consulting with colleagues helps define what is "reasonable." As defined in the APA Ethics Code, "the term *reasonable* means the prevailing professional judgment of psychologists engaged in similar activities in similar circumstances, given the knowledge the psychologist had or should have had at the time" (APA, 2002, p. 1062). In other words, reasonable decisions are based on prevailing professional judgment, which can be discovered through consultation with other professionals. Consultation with a colleague provides an operational definition of reasonable.

Practicing good ethics is not the same as preventing bad outcomes. The main reason to aspire to ethical excellence is to benefit the client, whereas the primary reason to practice liability risk management is to avoid harming the client. The secondary reason to provide liability risk management is to avoid harm to the clinician in the form of a malpractice action. From a professional liability risk-management perspective, consultation with a colleague makes it difficult for a plaintiff to prove a breach of a standard of care. In other words, "Reasonable clinicians protect themselves by protecting their patients" (Doverspike, 2004a, p. 210), and one of the best ways to protect the patient is to provide a reasonable standard of care.

Professional malpractice (often referred to as professional negligence) refers to an abrogation of a duty of care owed by a practitioner to a patient, as evidenced by a failure to exercise the degree of skill and care used by reasonable practitioners of similar qualifications in the same or similar circumstances. For a plaintiff to prevail in a professional liability lawsuit and collect damages in a court, the plaintiff's attorney must prove that the practitioner owed the patient a duty and that the practitioner's deviation from the standards of practice caused the patient's injury. The plaintiff's attorney must prove the "Four Ds" of malpractice: *duty* (that there existed a professional relationship that established a fiduciary duty to practice within a standard of care), *dereliction* of duty (that there was a breach of duty such as professional negligence and a failure to provide a reasonable standard of care), *damages* (that there were actual injuries or damages, which translates into dollars), and *direct* or proximate cause (that the damages or harm would not have occurred had it not been for the practitioner's negligence). Dereliction of duty can involve acts of commission (actions that harm a patient) or, more commonly, acts of omission (negligence or failure to perform actions that benefit a patient). One of the best ways to avoid dereliction of duty is to practice in a way that reasonable practitioners practice. A practitioner who obtains regular consultations is generally a practitioner who is being reasonable. Furthermore, because proof of professional negligence usually requires that an expert witness testify that the practitioner's performance was below a reasonable standard of care, the defendant practitioner who has already obtained collegial consultations is usually a practitioner who has already provided some proof that he or she was striving for a reasonable standard of care.

What are the two practices that R. L. Bednar (1991) and his colleagues recommend as ways "that will most dramatically reduce the chances of successful malpractice suits" (p. 59)? The two practices are *collegial consultations* and *good documentation* (record keeping). If your decisions and actions in a case are guided in part by consultation, be sure to document such consultation in your notes. Documentation of your consultation with a colleague demonstrates your careful consideration of the appropriate standards of care. In the worst-case scenario of a malpractice suit, your consultation and documentation will be your best evidence that you practiced within a reasonable standard of care. In his professional liability risk-management seminars, Harris (2004) gives a word of advice about asking for advice: "Don't ask for advice and then not follow it, unless you leave a documentary trail to show why a different decision was made." In other words, regardless of whether you follow the consultant's advice, document your decision-making process.

In my academic experience, which is based on more than a decade of teaching ethics and professional standards in doctoral clinical psychology and master's counseling training programs, I have been dismayed with how little attention the major textbooks devote to the actual ethical dilemmas with which most practitioners struggle in their day-to-day practices. With chapters ranging from values clarification and multiculturalism to scholarly research and publications, most of the major ethics textbooks devote relatively few pages to the areas of practice that affect practitioners the most.* This observation is consistent with Gibson and Pope's (1993) statement, "The low ratings that counselors give to published clinical and theoretical work suggests that authors of such work might consider why ethical aspects are not prominent in their publications or, if prominent, are not more useful as a source of guidance for practicing counselors" (p. 335). Gibson and Pope's observation is also consistent with Pope et al.'s (1987) earlier critique relevant to professional psychologists: "It is possible that research too rarely addresses ethical

---

* Perhaps one exception to these statements is Haas and Malouf's (2005) *Keeping Up the Good Work: A Practitioner's Guide to Mental Health Ethics* (4th ed.), which lives up to its subtitle as a practical handbook for practitioners.

concerns and standards of practice in a way that is useful for psychologists" (p. 1004). Given the low ratings that practicing mental health professions accord to scholarly research, perhaps the following discussion of common reasons that practitioners seek consultations will be more useful to professional psychologists and practicing counselors.

In my professional experience, which is based on providing ethics consultations as part of a professional ethics committee, there are some fairly predictable questions that practitioners often ask. Because my experience is based on professional experience and observations rather than formal surveys of empirical research, it may not be representative of the general population of practitioners. From a scientific perspective, I might be considered a participant-observer who has made observations of a self-selected sample of practitioners who have called their state professional association ethics committee seeking ethics consultations. Notwithstanding the limited generalizability of these observations, a review of some common reasons that practitioners seek consultations may benefit other practitioners who face similar situations. In this respect, the present review may be more beneficial than those suggested by the troublingly "low ratings accorded to published research" (Pope et al., 1987, p. 1004), by professional psychologists. Of course, there are no such things as "top 10 reasons" for seeking consultation, but there are several common scenarios that arise with predictable regularity. Based on some of the common scenarios that colleagues often encounter (Doverspike, 2001), the most common reasons for seeking ethics consultations include the following. The discussion of each of these topics is not exhaustive, but simply a highlight of a few points to consider in each area:

- Record retention, progress notes, and access to records
- Third-party requests for services
- Release of information and responding to subpoenas
- Release of raw test data and requests for test materials
- Dual relationships, including contemplated and unforeseeable relationships
- Couples counseling
- Child custody evaluations and other forensic evaluations
- Mandated reporting of suspected child abuse
- Discretionary duty to protect third parties from harm
- Termination of noncompliant or threatening clients
- Internet and electronic media
- Supervision, education, and training

- Reporting ethical violations of colleagues
- Responding to ethical violations in organizations
- Ethics and the law

Record Keeping

How long should you keep records? This is one of the most common ethics questions and perhaps the question with the most answers. Briefly, the answer depends on which ethical or legal standard you cite. As a starting point, the APA (2007) *Record Keeping Guidelines* specify the following:

> In the absence of a superceding requirement, psychologists may consider retaining full records until 7 years after the last date of service delivery for adults or until 3 years after a minor reaches the age of majority, whichever is later. (p. 10)

The above time limits were foreshadowed by a footnote in the earlier APA (1993) *Record Keeping Guidelines*, which stated that,

> if the specialty guidelines should be revised, a simple 7 year requirement for the retention of the complete record is preferred, which would be a more stringent requirement than any existing state statute. (p. 985)

It should be pointed out that the 1993 APA standard was far less stringent than current prevailing standards that have evolved since the 1993 guidelines were published. For example, there is at least one recommendation that the record be maintained for 10 years following termination of treatment (Behnke, Preis, & Bates, 1998), with record retention for 10 years after a minor has turned 21.

Another recent development in record retention involves the federal HIPAA regulations. Although HIPAA regulations do not explicitly specify a period of retention for mental health records, the phrase "previous six years" occurs in several places in the federal regulations. For this reason, one might logically infer that 7 years would be a conservative retention period for a record assuming that there are no disclosures made from the record and that there are no requests for access to the record. Such an inference operates under these assumptions (i.e., that there are no disclosures made from the record and no requests made for access to the record) because the documentation requirements for such requests would themselves have the effect of extending the retention period indefinitely. Implicit in the HIPAA regulations is the assumption that documentation of access and requests for records must continue to be maintained as long as there are "requests for access by patients." If the HIPAA compliant provider receives a "request for access by patients" every 5 years, for example, then it is possible that the designated record set would have to be maintained indefinitely. In other words, it is within the realm of possibilities that the records would have to be maintained ad infinitum.

A 7-year retention period for the complete record is generally consistent with trends in the ethics literature (Koocher & Keith-Spiegel, 1998). In the sixth edition of their multidisciplinary ethics textbook, G. Corey, M. Corey, and Callanan (2003) recommend a minimum of a 7-year retention period with an additional retention period for a summary of the record:

> Providers have an obligation to keep records for a minimum of 7 years following the termination of a client. Organization policy often prescribes guidelines for maintaining records, including a time frame. In the absence of such laws, the general recommendation is that complete records should be kept for a minimum of 3 years after the last contact with a client. Records, or a summary, should then be maintained for an additional 12 years before disposal. (p. 167)

The G. Corey et al. (2003) recommendations follow the general model of the earlier APA (1993) *Record Keeping Guidelines*, which have been superceded by the APA (2007) *Record Keeping Guidelines*. In the seventh edition of their ethics textbook, however, G. Corey et al. (2007) offer much less specificity by stating, "Depending on one's place of practice and the types of records kept, clients' records must be maintained for the period of time required by relevant federal, state, and local laws" (p. 174).

For adults, a reasonable standard would be to keep the complete record for a period of at least 7 years, and keep either the complete record or a summary of the record for a total of 15 years after the last date service was rendered. To provide greater access by the patient and to maintain a higher standard of care, a HIPAA compliant provider would be advised to keep the complete record or a summary for at least 15 years after the last date of a request for access by the patient. To achieve the highest standard, keep the full record as long as is reasonably possible (Behnke et al., 1998).

Record Keeping and Progress Notes

How much information should you put into your progress notes? This question should be answered within the context of the more general question: What has to be kept in records? The APA (1987) *General Guidelines for Providers of Psychological Services* state that case notes minimally include dates and types of services as well as any "significant actions taken" (p. 717). The more current APA (2007) *Record Keeping Guidelines* specify the following:

> Identifying data (e.g., name, client ID number); contact information (e.g., phone number, address, next of kin); fees and billing information; where appropriate, guardianship or conservatorship status; documentation of informed consent or assent for treatment (Ethics Code 3.10); documentation of waivers of confidentiality and authorization or consent for release of information (Ethics Code 4.05); documentation of any mandated disclosure of confidential information (e.g., report of child abuse, release secondary to a court order); presenting complaint, diagnosis, or basis for request for services; plan for services, updated as appropriate (e.g., treatment plan, supervision plan, intervention schedule, community interventions, consultation contracts); health and developmental history. (p. 6)

In addition to the preceding basic information that should be included in every client's record, the APA (2007) guidelines also specify the following information to be included in the record for each substantive contact with a client:

> Date of service and duration of session; types of services (e.g., consultation, assessment, treatment, training); nature of professional intervention or contact (e.g., treatment modalities, referral, letters, e-mail, phone contacts); formal or informal assessment of client status. (p. 7)

Depending on the circumstances, the record may also include other specific information as delineated by the APA (2007) *Record Keeping Guidelines*:

> Client responses or reactions to professional interventions; current risk factors in relation to dangerousness to self or others; other

treatment modalities employed such as medication or biofeedback treatment; emergency interventions (e.g., specially scheduled sessions, hospitalizations); plans for future interventions; information describing the qualitative aspects of the professional/ client interaction; prognosis; assessment or summary data (e.g., psychological testing, structured interviews, behavioral ratings, client behavior logs); consultations with or referrals to other professionals; case-related telephone, mail, and e-mail contacts; relevant cultural and sociopolitical factors. (p. 7)

State laws may differ from APA requirements. For example, licensed psychologists in Georgia must consider Chapter 510-5-.04 (Maintenance and Retention of Records) of the 2004 Georgia Supplemental Code of Conduct,* which specifies that professional psychological records shall include the following:

(1) identifying data, (2) dates of services, (3) types of services, (4) fees, (5) assessments, (6) treatment plan, (7) consultation, (8) summary reports and/or testing reports, (9) supporting data as may be required, and (10) any release of information obtained. (p. 53)

Many state licensing boards do not even specify a record retention period or the content required in the records, in which case practitioners licensed under those boards are usually advised to consider other applicable legal and professional standards. For example, Section (2[C] Unprofessional conduct . . .) of Chapter 135-7-.03 (Confidentiality) of the Rules of Georgia Composite Board of Professional Counselors, Social Workers, and Marriage and Family Therapists does not specify a length of record retention nor contents that are required in client records. In fact, there is only one reference to client "records" in Section (2[C]) of Chapter 135-7-.03, which reads as follows:

(2) Unprofessional conduct includes but is not limited to the following: . . . (c) failing to store or dispose of client records in a way that maintains confidentiality, and when providing any client with access to that client's records, failing to protect the confidences of other persons contained in that record. (p. 40)

---

* The Georgia record retention rules were in the process of being revised at the time of publication of this book. (See also pages 176 and 183.)

How much information should you put into your progress notes? Think of it as a business decision of how much time and energy are needed to justify your desired level of protection (Bennett et al., 1997). Psychologist/attorney Eric Harris has advised that progress notes should not only explain "what you did and why you did it" but, just as importantly, they should explain "what you didn't do and why you didn't do it" (Harris, 2004; Stromberg et al., 1988). Remember that good record keeping provides the first indication to a reviewer that your treatment meets minimum standards of care.

In discussing the client record as a tool in risk management, Piazza and Yeager (1991) recommend that psychologists "not write anything in the client's records that you would not want a client's lawyer to read" (p. 344). Doverspike (1999b) suggests that you not only write your notes the way you would like to read them in court, but write them the way you would like *someone else* to read them in court. An even more paranoid documentation strategy is suggested by Gutheil (1980) who recommends, "In writing progress notes, trainees are urged to hallucinate on their shoulder the image of a hostile prosecuting attorney who might preside at the trial in which their records are subpoenaed" (p. 481). A less paranoid strategy would be to not only write your notes in a risk-managed way that you would want your client's attorney to read them in court, but also write them in a user-friendly way that you would want your client to read them in your office (Doverspike, 2006c, p. 14).

Access to Records

Does the patient always have a right to his or her records? The answers are "Yes and no." For psychologists, APA (2002) Ethical Standard 4.05 (Disclosures) states, "(a) Psychologists may disclose confidential information with the appropriate consent of the organizational client, the individual client/patient, or another legally authorized person on behalf of the client/patient unless prohibited by law" (p. 1066). For counselors, ACA (2005) Section B.6.d. (Client Access) states, "Counselors provide reasonable access to records and copies of records when requested by competent clients" (p. 8). In other words, the client/patient has the right to request a disclosure of confidential information that is contained in his or her record.

In general, the only other stated exception to these requirements involves withholding records for nonpayment of services in situations in which the records are needed for nonemergencies. Under APA (2002) Ethical Standard 6.03 (Withholding Records for Nonpayment),

"Psychologists may not withhold records under their control that are requested and needed for a client's/patient's emergency treatment solely because payment has not been received" (p. 1068). Similarly, ACA Section B.6.d. (Client Access) states, "Counselors limit the access of clients to their records, or portions of their records, only when there is compelling evidence that such access would cause harm to the client. Counselors document the request of clients and the rationale for withholding some or all of the record in the files of clients" (p. 8). However, keep in mind that in the adjudication of an ethics complaint related to failure to release records to a client, most state licensing boards are concerned more about protecting clients' rights than therapists' incomes.

The APA and ACA ethical standards are consistent with HIPAA federal regulations that are designed to protect patients' rights. For example, the HIPAA Privacy Rule gives patients certain rights of access to, and knowledge of, how their records will be used and disclosed. With limited exception, the Privacy Rule gives patients the right to inspect and obtain a copy of protected health information in the record. In addition to protecting the patient's right to access, HIPAA regulations also protect the patient's rights to amend records, to consent to disclosure of the record, to obtain an accounting of disclosure from the records, and to request restrictions on the use and disclosure of protected health information in the record.

With respect to state laws, many states provide protection of patients' rights similar to those specified in the Privacy Rule, in which case the state laws preempt HIPAA and will apply in place of the Privacy Rule. In states that provide less protection than HIPAA, the Privacy Rule prevails. For example, for health care providers in Georgia, O.C.G.A. § 31-33-2(a)(2) (Furnishing Copy of Records to Patient, Provider, or Other Authorized Person, 2006) specifies, "Upon written request from the patient or a person authorized to have access to the patient's record under a health care power of attorney for such patient, the provider having custody and control of the patient's record shall furnish a complete and current copy of that record, in accordance with the provisions of this Code section." However, there is one statutory exception to this requirement in the case of patients for whom a disclosure may be harmful to the patient. Chapter 31-33-2(c) specifies that, "If the provider reasonably determines that disclosure of the record to the patient will be detrimental to the physical or mental health of the patient, the provider may refuse to furnish the record; however, upon such refusal, the patient's record shall be furnished to any other provider designated by the patient." Although this statute is often cited as being applicable to licensed health care providers, it is important to note the following exception specified by Chapter 31-33-4 (Mental Health Records, 1985): "The provisions of this chapter shall not apply to psychiatric, psychological, or other mental health records of a patient." Nevertheless, this law continues to be cited as statutorily creating a patient's right to access of his or her record, unless such access to the record would be reasonably determined to cause harm to the patient.

Who owns the record? This question is a legal question rather than an ethics question. In general, the provider owns the record, although the patient owns the right of access to the record. For medical records, Chapter 31-33-2(b) of the 1981 Georgia Code originally specified, "Nothing in this chapter shall be construed as granting to a patient any right of ownership in the records, as such records are owned by and are the property of the provider." However, in compliance with federal HIPAA regulations, Chapter 31-33-2(b) of the 2006 Georgia Code was revised as follows:

> Any record requested under subsection (a) of this Code section shall within 30 days of the receipt of a request for records be furnished to the patient, any other provider designated by the patient, any person authorized by paragraph (2) of subsection (a) of this Code section to request a patient's or deceased patient's medical records, or any other person designated by the patient. Such record request shall be accompanied by: (1) An authorization in compliance with the federal Health Insurance Portability and Accountability Act of 1996, 42 U.S.C. Section 1320d-2, et seq., and regulations implementing such act; and (2) A signed written authorization as specified in subsection (d) of this Code section.

In plain English, the provider is the custodian and guardian of the record whereas the patient or his or her legal representative has the right of access to the record. Because the ownership of records is essentially a legal matter, it is recommended that the practitioner consult with legal counsel on a case-by-case basis when such questions arise.

Who owns the records of a deceased person? It is often said that the psychotherapeutic privilege survives death, meaning that the confidentiality of psychotherapeutic communications is protected regardless of whether or not the patient is living. Like many ethical responsibilities, maintaining confidentiality is not based merely on the amount of time that has elapsed since the communications were made. Ethical responsibilities are usually intertwined with legal requirements, and the right of access to the mental health records of deceased patients may vary from state to state. Because state laws preempt HIPAA regulations in cases in which state laws provide the patient with greater protection of privacy or greater access to records, an understanding of specific state laws is required. For example, according to O.C.G.A. § 31-33-2, the following persons may request medical records in Georgia if the patient is deceased:

(A) The executor, administrator, or temporary administrator for the decedent's estate if such person has been appointed;

(B) If an executor, administrator, or temporary administrator for the decedent's estate has not been appointed, by the surviving spouse;

(C) If there is no surviving spouse, by any surviving child; and

(D) If there is no surviving child, any parent.

The statutory language of O.C.G.A. § 31-33-2 (i.e., "such request may be made") permits certain designated persons to make requests for records, although the statute does not require that the custodian release the records. Furthermore, notwithstanding the statutory right to request the medical records of a deceased patient in Georgia, it is important to remember that the provisions of Chapter 31-33-2 do not apply to psychiatric, psychological, or other mental health records of a patient. For this reason, the prudent practitioner is often advised to have the person requesting such records to seek a court order. As with any legal question, always consult an attorney for legal advice before making a decision.

Third-Party Requests

Do you have to give the client a written report of assessment results? The answer may depend on what was understood and agreed upon in advance during the discussion of informed consent. In general, an individual or organizational client is entitled to a report of assessment results. This type of situation typically arises in the case of Independent Consultative Examinations, which fall under the general heading of Third-Party Requests for Services. APA Ethical Standard 3.07 (Third-Party Requests for Services) specifies the following:

> When psychologists agree to provide services to a person or entity at the request of a third party, psychologists attempt to clarify at the outset of the service the nature of the relationship with all individuals or organizations involved. This clarification includes

the role of the psychologist (e.g., therapist, consultant, diagnostician, or expert witness), an identification of who is the client, the probable uses of the services provided or the information obtained, and the fact that there may be limits to confidentiality. (p. 1065)

In Third-Party Requests for Services, the referring organizational client receives an oral or written report of assessment results of the person being evaluated. However, before undergoing the evaluation, the person being evaluated gives advance informed consent that includes an understanding and agreement of whether he or she will receive a copy of the assessment results. Primary prevention of ethical problems usually goes back to the clarity with which informed consent has been established. Preventing ethical problems from developing in third-party consultative exams can be facilitated through an informed consent process involving identification of the client, clarification of the psychologist's role, specification of the services provided, and explanation of the limits of confidentiality.

In third-party requests for services, the person being evaluated is not the client. For this reason, the person being evaluated may or may not be entitled to receive a written report of assessment results unless such a disclosure is permitted by the organizational client. APA Ethical Standard 9.10 (Explaining Assessment Results) specifies the following:

Regardless of whether the scoring and interpretation are done by psychologists, by employees or assistants, or by automated or other outside services, psychologists take reasonable steps to ensure that explanations of results are given to the individual or designated representative unless the nature of the relationship precludes provision of an explanation of results (such as in some organizational consulting, preemployment or security screenings, and forensic evaluations), and this fact has been clearly explained to the person being assessed in advance. (p. 1072)

The APA Ethical Standard does not state that a written psychological report must be prepared, but it does state that the person being evaluated is entitled to "an explanation of the results" *unless this is precluded by prior agreement.* If you do not plan to prepare a written report of assessment results, make sure that you have clearly explained this to the person in advance. One bit of practical advice is to always prepare a written report of assessment results and inform the client in advance that there will be a charge for the report. If the person being evaluated is not entitled to a written report of an evaluation that is requested by a third-party organizational client, make sure that you have obtained and documented the evaluated person's understanding and agreement in advance. In other words, prevent an ethical problem by managing the person's expectations in advance. Establish realistic expectations on the part of the organizational client and on the part of the person being evaluated at the request of the organizational client. A sample informed consent form is contained on the CD-ROM accompanying this book.

Release of Information

What should you do if you receive a subpoena? This common question is just one example of the many types of questions that are asked about requests for confidential information. Here are some other typical questions and variations on the same theme: What should you do if you receive a subpoena or request for production of records from one of your former clients for whom you provided marriage counseling? Does a release of information always have to be in writing? Should you fax or email confidential information to an insurance company to obtain payment of a claim? Who owns and controls the privilege of a deceased person's records?

In response to the question about how to respond to a subpoena, the answer is complicated by the fact that there are actually three types of subpoenas, two of which can be used to order a person to appear in court as a witness to testify and the third type of which can be used to order a person to testify at a deposition. A *Subpoena to Appear* is used to order a witness to appear in court, but not necessarily to bring documents or records to court. A *Subpoena to Appear and Produce* is used to order a witness to bring along certain documents when the witness appears in court to testify. A *Subpoena to Take a Deposition* is used to order a person to testify at a deposition at which the sworn testimony of a witness is taken outside of court. Regardless of the type of subpoena, remember that a subpoena compels a *response* but does not compel a *disclosure* (Bennett et al., 1996). In many cases, the proper first response to a subpoena is to assert the privilege. Remar and Hubert (1996) provide an analysis of appropriate ways of responding to requests for production, subpoenas, and court orders. The following guidelines are recommended by Remar and Hubert:

An MHP [mental health practitioner] who receives a subpoena should immediately notify the patient or the patient's attorney. If the patient executes a written authorization for release of the information, the MHP may produce the records. If the MHP is unable to obtain the patient's express authorization, then the MHP should, within 10 days after the service of the subpoena or on or before the time specified in the subpoena for compliance if such time is less than 10 days after service, deliver to the attorney designated in the subpoena a written objection to inspection or copying of the records. (p. 117)

A footnote in Remar and Hubert's recommendation states that in federal courts, the time period for a response is 14 days. Samples of letters for responding to a subpoena are contained in the *GPA Psychologists' Toolbox: Strategies for Building and Maintaining a Successful Private Practice* (Sauls et al., 2001) as well as the CD-ROM accompanying this book. Finally, because a subpoena is a legal document requiring a legal response, always consult with an attorney before responding to a subpoena.

Regarding questions related to requests for records of a former client for whom you previously provided couples counseling or marital therapy, the general rule is to manage all of your clients' expectations in advance through the process of informed consent. Clients undergoing couples counseling are informed in advance that any subsequent requests for records will require the signed, written authorization of both participants in the couples counseling. In the case of clients who request treatment while in the middle of a divorce proceeding, Ellis (2006) notes that some clinicians ask the client to sign an agreement stating that he or she will not subpoena the therapist pursuant to divorce of custody-related matters. Although such an agreement does not waive the client's right to request records or subpoena the therapist, such an agreement does represent an attempt to manage the psychotherapy client's expectations from the outset. A related matter that must be addressed as part of the informed consent discussion involves the legal concept of privileged communication. According to G. Corey et al. (2007), "the legal concept of privileged communication does *not* apply to group counseling, couples counseling, marital and family therapy, or child and adolescent therapy" (p. 211). Because privileged communication statutes in some states do not apply to communications in couples and family therapy, it may be best for couples counselors and marital therapists to assume that such communications are not privileged. Couples counselors, marital therapists, and group therapists are advised to inform their clients of the lack of legal privilege concerning disclosures made in the presence of third parties (B. S. Anderson, 1996).

Informed consent in couples therapy is important not only in terms of how and when information will be disclosed to third parties outside the sessions, but also in terms of how and when information disclosed privately by one partner to the therapist will be disclosed by the therapist to the other partner within couples therapy sessions. Individuals in couples therapy often disclose information privately to therapists in several ways, such as during an individual session, by a telephone call, or even in a letter. There are generally three ways marital and family therapists handle information disclosed individually by a client, including (a) *complete confidentiality*, in which the therapist does not disclose in a couples or family session any information given to the therapist by individuals in private sessions; (b) *no confidentiality*, in which the therapist discloses all information given to the therapist privately by any individual; and (c) *limited confidentiality*, in which the therapist uses professional judgment and reserves the right to disclose information in light of the best interests of the couple or family. The limited confidentiality policy offers the most flexibility and allows the greatest latitude in professional judgment than either of the two more extreme positions. In general, most marital and family therapists refuse to keep information secret that was shared individually with the therapist because secrets can otherwise encourage hidden agendas, contribute to triangulation, and create ethical dilemmas for the therapist. Regardless of which of the previous policies the therapist prefers, the most important ethical considerations involve creating realistic client expectations in advance through the initial informed consent discussion and through the ongoing process of communication with the clients.

Regarding questions related to the release of a deceased client's records, it is important to consult with your attorney before taking any action because there are often conflicts between state laws and federal regulations. Under Subsection C (Personal Representatives of Deceased Patients) of Section VII (Uses and Disclosures Involving Personal Representatives), the American Psychological Association Practice Organization (APAPO; 2002, p. 17) *Getting Ready for HIPAA: A Primer for Psychologists* provides the following interpretation of HIPAA standards related to the records of a deceased patient:

> The psychologist must treat the legal representative of a deceased patient as the patient with respect to PHI that is relevant to the representative's representation (letting the personal representative

exercise the privacy rights that a patient would normally exercise [e.g., receiving notice, consenting to disclosure, having access to records and the right to amend]).

However, because state laws may preempt federal HIPAA regulations in cases in which state laws provide the patient with greater protection of privacy or increased access to his or her records, the preceding HIPAA standard may come into direct conflict with the laws of some states that do not statutorily specify a waiver of privilege of a deceased client's records. For example, as cited in Remar and Hubert (1996, p. 97), "a 1994 amendment to the [Georgia] Mental Health Code provides that a copy of the record may be released to the legal representative of a deceased patient's estate, *except in the case of privileged matters* [italics added]" (1996, p. 97). It is for this reason that in some states it is sometimes said, "Patient privilege survives death." In any situation in which there is a conflict between state laws and federal regulations, particularly when such statutes are being continually revised and updated, always consult with an attorney before responding to a request for production of records.

**Release of
Test Data**

Ethical Standard 2.02b (Competence and Appropriate Use of Assessments and Interventions) of the 1992 APA *Ethical Principles* cautioned psychologists against misuse of assessment techniques, interventions, and test results by unqualified persons. As specified in Ethical Standard 2.02b, this precaution included "refraining from releasing raw test results or raw data to persons, other than to patients or clients as appropriate, who are not qualified to use such information" (APA, 1992, p. 1603). The wording of the 1992 standard often resulted in psychologists refusing to release raw scores to attorneys, school teachers, and others even when the client's request was accompanied by a signed written authorization. Partly in response to the controversy, the American Psychological Association (1996) produced a flow-chart for ethical decision making in responding to court ordered disclosures, particularly as these relate to requests for psychological test raw data. Particularly in the field of neuropsychology, the release of psychological data to nonexperts was a topic that received considerable scholarly debate (Barth, 2000; Lees-Haley & Courtney, 2000a, 2000b; Shapiro, 2000; Tranel, 1994, 2000) before the publication of the 2002 APA Ethical Principles.

In contrast to the 1992 standard, the 2002 Ethical Standard 9.04a (Release of Test Data) clarifies that, "Pursuant to a client/patient release, psychologists provide test data to the client/patient or other persons identified in the release" (p. 1071). The only exceptions to this requirement are when test data may be withheld to protect the patient or others from substantial harm or to protect against misuse or misrepresentation of the data or the test. The 2002 Ethical Standard 9.04 (Release of Test Data) specifically states:

> Psychologists may refrain from releasing test data to protect a client/patient or others from substantial harm or misuse or misrepresentation of the data or the test, recognizing that in many instances release of confidential information under these circumstances is regulated by law. (pp. 1071-1072)

In dissecting the previous ethical standard, there are six grounds upon which a psychologist may ethically refuse to release psychological test data in response to a valid authorization signed by the client. Psychologists are advised to release test data in response to a valid authorization unless at least one of the following provisions is met:

- To protect client from substantial harm
- To protect others from substantial harm
- To protect from misuse of the data
- To protect from misuse of the test
- To protect from misrepresentation of the data
- To protect from misrepresentation of the test

In the absence of a client/patient release, APA (2002) Ethical Standard 9.04(b) specifies that psychologists may provide test data "only as required by law or court order" (p. 1072). These standards relate to the release of *test data*, which are defined as "those portions of test materials that include client/patient responses" (p. 1071). These standards do not relate to the release of test *protocols*, which are otherwise protected by law, contractual obligations, and security requirements. APA Ethical Standard 9.11 (Maintaining Test Security) requires that "psychologists make reasonable efforts to maintain the integrity and security of test materials and other assessment techniques, consistent with law and contractual obligations, and in a manner that permits adherence to this Ethics Code" (p. 1072). Test materials include "manuals, instruments, protocols, and test questions or stimuli" (p. 1072).

According to APA Ethical Standard 9.04(a), "The term *test data* refers to raw and scaled scores, client/patient responses to test questions or stimuli, and psychologists' notes and recordings concerning client/patient statements and behavior during an examination" (p. 1071). Based on the APA definitions, Table 5 (below) illustrates some of the differences between test data and test materials.

Psychologists are advised to release "test data" or other information requested by the client/patient to the person identified in the release, unless to do so would cause (a) substantial harm to the client/patient or others or (b) misuse or misinterpretation of the data or test. When a psychologist is faced with the ethical dilemma of whether to release test data, the psychologist should consider whether the release of the test data would result in one of the following six adverse consequences specified in Ethical Standard 9.04: (a) harm to the client/patient, (b) harm to others, (c) misuse of the data, (d) misinterpretation of the data, (e) misuse of the test, and (f) misinterpretation of the test. In the presence of a valid request for release of information, the psychologist would be advised to release the test data unless one of the aforementioned conditions is reasonably foreseeable. In the absence of a valid authorization for release, provide the information only as required by law or court order. Although there may be some basis for withholding records for nonpayment of services in situations that do not involve emergencies, such a practice may be unwise and may in fact conflict with some of the federal HIPAA provisions that protect the patient's right of access to his or her records.

Table 5: Difference Between Test Data and Test Materials

Test Data	Test Materials
Raw scores	Manuals
Responses to test questions or stimuli	Instruments
Psychologist's notes and recordings of statements and behavior	Protocols
Portions of test materials that include client responses	Test questions or stimuli

Dual Relationships

Is it ethical to provide therapy to a member of [fill in the name of your organization]? This question is a variation on the theme of other common questions: Is it okay to provide therapy to a member of your club, church, temple, or tennis team? The ethical shades of gray may depend on the size of the organization, your degree of involvement with the organization, your potential client's degree of involvement with the organization, and your degree of involvement with your potential client within the organization. Questions in the gray areas of ethics, such as those involving contemplated nonsexual dual relationships, can often be approached by using an ethical decision-making model or problem-solving approach to ethics (Gottlieb, 1993).

Is it ethical for you to hire a former client to do work at [fill in the name of your place of employment]? Subtle ethical conflicts often become more obvious when one changes the context of the question, such as the following: It is okay to hire a former student to do some work in your office? Is it okay to hire a former student to do some work in your home? In Georgia, the best way to answer these questions is to refer to the last line of Chapter 510-5-.05(2) of the Georgia Code of Conduct (2004). With reference to the topic of Prohibited Dual Relationships, this section states:

> The psychologist, in interacting with a client, former client, supervisee, employee, research participant, student, or others with whom the psychologist has or had authority within the previous 24 months, shall not (a) engage in any verbal or physical behavior toward the individual which is sexually seductive, demeaning, or harassing; or (b) engage in sexual intercourse or other physical intimacies with the individual; or (c) enter into a financial or other potentially exploitative relationship with the individual. (p. 46)

Practical advice in plain English: Don't hire former clients to work in your home or office.

Another area of dual relationships involves client special requests. For example, assume that your client invited you to [fill in the name of the event]. What should you do? Of course, this is another variation on the theme of a dual relationship. Whereas prohibited dual relationships are always unethical, there are some dual relationships and boundary crossings that are not unethical. Gutheil and Gabbard (1993) distinguish between *boundary crossings* (changes in role that benefit a client) and *boundary violations* (changes in role that harm or exploit a client). As discussed previously in Chapter Three (Managing Boundaries), a boundary crossing is a departure from commonly accepted practices that could potentially benefit a client, whereas a boundary violation is a serious breach that results in harm or exploitation of a client. Boundary crossings involve changes in the therapist's role, while boundary violations involve exploitation of the client. The problem with boundary crossings is that they increase the risk of boundary violations (the so-called "slippery slope" phenomenon).

Baird (2001) has offered the following guidelines for therapists when responding to a patient request to step outside of the traditional therapeutic framework: (a) Ask yourself how the patient's request can be addressed within a traditional therapeutic framework; (b) consider the ways in which the request may reflect a desire on the part of the patient for the therapist to meet the needs of the patient which were unmet by important people in the patient's life; (c) interpret (rather than gratify) the request whenever appropriate; and (d) always consult with a colleague before stepping outside traditional therapeutic boundaries.

Couples Counseling

Is it ethical to provide couples counseling for a client for whom you have also provided individual psychotherapy? Is it ethical to provide individual therapy for a client for whom you have provided couples counseling? These are questions that are sometimes asked by therapists who have not yet clarified the boundaries of their own practices. Is it ethical for a client to shift from individual therapy to couples therapy? Woodsfellow (2004) provides an ethical analysis of what is sometimes described as *consecutive therapy,* which involves a client shifting from individual psychotherapy to couples therapy with the same therapist. There are essentially three types of consecutive shifts, although the third type occurs only after an initial shift has taken place in what originally began as couples therapy. The first and perhaps most common type of consecutive shift, hereafter referred to as Type I, occurs when a client shifts from individual therapy to couples therapy as described by Woodsfellow. This type of shift essentially involves role-blending in a foreseeable consecutive dual relationship, based on the criteria previously discussed in Chapter Three (Managing Boundaries) in this book. The second type of shift (Type II) occurs when a client shifts from couples therapy to individual therapy with the same therapist after the other partner in therapy has either dropped out or terminated therapy. This type of shift may occur, for example, if one of the partners in a relationship decides to leave the relationship and the other partner decides to continue seeing the same therapist on an individual basis. The third and least frequent type of shift (Type III) occurs only when the partner who dropped out of therapy decides to resume either individual or couples therapy with the same therapist who has been continuing to provide individual therapy for the other party. Although each of these scenarios involves different dynamics and different ethical implications, all of these scenarios involve a dual relationship, role-blending, and the risk of possible loss of objectivity or loss of effectiveness on the part of the therapist. Each of these types of consecutive shifts is discussed briefly below.

As Woodsfellow correctly points out, the Type I consecutive shift is so prevalent in the mental health professions that it could even be considered within an acceptable standard of care. Furthermore, there are no ethical prohibitions against consecutive therapy in the ethics codes of any of the mental health professions, including the American Psychiatric Association, the American Psychological Association, the American Counseling Association, the American Association for Marriage and Family Therapy, and the National Association of Social Workers. Nevertheless, although the practice may not be ethically prohibited, it is ethically problematic. As Woodsfellow observes, "the potential problems with consecutive therapy are quite substantial" (p. 19). In addition to addressing the initial transition issues related to confidentiality of material from previous individual sessions and informed consent regarding the new arrangements, there are also potential complications related to maintaining therapeutic neutrality in the face of shifting loyalties. For example, even if the therapist could maintain complete therapeutic neutrality, there is no guarantee that each of the partners would perceive the therapist as being neutral in the new role. Because this scenario is so fraught with ethical pitfalls, Woodsfellow strongly advises against consecutive therapy.

The Type II consecutive shift is also a relatively common practice among therapists, with perhaps greater justification and more prevalence than the Type I shift. The Type II shift is supported by the argument that it is often easier, more expedient, and more economical for a client to continue individual therapy with a therapist who has already established a relationship with the client. However, ease, expediency, and economy are not necessarily ethical justifications for actions. The therapist must be guided by the best interests of the client(s), which in this case would include the former client as well as the active client. One of the main problems of the Type II consecutive shift is that it essentially prevents one partner (i.e., the one who drops out prematurely) from being able to return to couples therapy in a manner that is not biased by the therapist's ongoing individual relationship with the other partner. In other words, the Type II consecutive shift is not ethically prohibited but neither is it ethically justified. If a therapist is willing to shift to individual therapy after one of the partners drops out of couples therapy, then advance informed consent *with both parties* becomes crucial because one of the parties may be thereby forgoing the opportunity to resume couples therapy at a later point in time. I recall that one of the first ethics committees investigations in which I participated involved a complaint from a former client who alleged that his former marital therapist had not allowed him to return to couples counseling with his wife who had shifted to individual therapy with the same therapist after the husband had prematurely terminated treatment. The ethics investigation focused primarily on the issues of professional competence, informed consent, and role-clarification. The ethical issue of competence was addressed first by determining whether the therapist had education, training, and supervised experience in conducting marital therapy. The ethical issues of informed consent and role-clarification were addressed by determining whether the therapist had clarified role expectations in advance as part of the informed consent discussion at the outset of therapy and again at the time that the consecutive shift occurred. At a minimum, the therapist would have been ethically obligated to have informed both partners of the therapist's policies for handling interruptions in therapy, premature termination of therapy, and changes in role expectations related to consecutive shift.

The Type III consecutive shift refers to what is sometimes described as an "ethical no-brainer." The shift occurs only when the partner who dropped out of therapy decides to resume either individual or, more commonly, couples therapy with the same therapist who has been continuing to provide individual therapy for the other party. The Type III shift is considered an ethical no-brainer because the scenario makes it virtually impossible for the therapist to maintain therapeutic neutrality and effectiveness with both parties when the alliance has shifted not once but twice. Because this type of shift is much more problematic than either of the preceding types, therapists are strongly advised to avoid it. Of course, one way to avoid this type of shift is to avoid the Type II shift, which sets the stage in the first place. If a therapist is truly providing couples therapy, then the best interests of the couple are of primary importance. If one partner terminates treatment, then there is no couple to treat. It may be a matter of convenience that the therapist continues providing therapy to one partner after the other partner has dropped out, but it is not necessarily good ethical practice.

Child Custody
Evaluations

Is it unethical to conduct a child custody evaluation if the child is in your own child's class at school? This scenario is a variation on the more general theme of a similar question: Is it unethical to perform a forensic evaluation on an individual who is a member of your child or family member's club, sports team, or Sunday School class? Is it unethical for you to testify as an expert witness regarding the parental fitness of one of your psychotherapy clients who is involved in child custody litigation? You probably already know the answers to these questions if you are familiar with the *Guidelines for Child Custody Evaluations in Divorce Proceedings* (APA, 1994). As a general response to these types of questions, psychologists are advised to avoid performing multiple and potentially conflicting roles in forensic matters (Greenberg & Shuman, 1997).

APA (2002) Ethical Standard 10.02b (Therapy Involving Couples or Families) states, "If it becomes apparent that psychologists may be called on to perform potentially conflicting roles (such as family therapist and then witness for one party in divorce proceedings), psychologists take reasonable steps to clarify and modify, or withdraw from, roles appropriately" (p. 1073). More specifically, the APA *Guidelines for Child Custody Evaluations in Divorce Proceedings* state:

> Psychologists generally avoid conducting a child custody evaluation in a case in which the psychologist served in a therapeutic role for the child or his or her immediate family or has had other involvement that may compromise the psychologist's objectivity. (p. 678)

If you have perceived mixed loyalties in a forensic case, you should assume that you will be cross-examined on this matter in court. Here's some practical advice in plain English: Avoid conducting forensic services involving persons with whom you have had a prior therapeutic or other perceived conflicting relationship. At the same time, avoid providing therapeutic services for persons with whom you have had a prior forensic relationship or other perceived conflicting relationship. In other words, avoid the unethical blending of therapeutic and forensic roles (Greenberg & Shuman, 1997; Harris, 2004; Younggren, 2006).

The area of child custody is so fraught with anger and blame that, if you are going to conduct custody evaluations, you should expect that a lawsuit or licensing board complaint will eventually be filed against you. Your best defense will be based on showing how you have been an objective and conscientious forensic evaluator who followed the "Top 10" rules of a forensic evaluator (Doverspike, 2005b). These rules include the following commonsense guidelines: (a) Do not have a prior conflict of interest with any of the referring parties or litigants; (b) do not blur therapeutic and forensic roles; (c) do have competence in performing evaluations in the areas required for the assessment; (d) do manage expectations by engaging in a process of adequate informed consent with all parties prior to the evaluation; (e) do document the process of informed consent; (f) do conduct a thorough evaluation consistent with professional standards; (g) do evaluate both parents and child(ren); (h) do write a report that can withstand scrutiny by an expert psychologist; (i) do clarify any unreliability of the data or findings; and (j) do limit the scope of your testimony to those matters for which you have established a reasonable empirical foundation. In other words, demonstrate that you maintained an appropriate standard by following guidelines such as the APA (1994) *Guidelines for Child Custody Evaluations in Divorce Proceedings*.

Mandated Reporting

Do you have to report child abuse if you are not sure it occurred? What if the abuse was not reported to you by the child? What if you suspect abuse but it is denied by the child? What if the victim of the abuse is now an adult? What if the perpetrator of abuse is your client? These questions are some examples of some of the most frequently encountered ethics questions related to the mandatory reporting of suspected abuse. Mandated reporting laws govern the reporting of reasonably suspected abuse of a minor child, elder person, or disabled or vulnerable adult. In my experience providing ethics consultations, the number of questions that I receive on the topic of mandated reporting are surpassed only by technical questions related to record keeping and access to confidential records. At first glance, the large number of phone calls is somewhat surprising in view of the fact that mandated reporting statutes are so clear-cut. However, Kalichman and Craig (1991) have found that clinicians are often hesitant to report suspected abuse unless they are fairly certain that abuse has occurred. In addition, clinicians may decide not to report suspected abuse due to their concerns about the negative impact their reporting may have on the therapeutic relationship (Kalichman & Craig, 1991). As a general rule, mental health professionals generally do not have as much familiarity or frequency of reporting as do personnel in educational settings, legal and law enforcement, and social service agencies.

The most common mandated reporting questions relate to suspected abuse of children rather than elder or vulnerable adults. In addition, questions related to mandated reporting often arise during child custody evaluations, sometimes because of actual child abuse and sometimes because of one parent's allegations of abuse by the other parent designed to place the other parent in an unfavorable position of having to defend such complaints. This statement is not meant to minimize the seriousness of child abuse or to suggest that divorcing parents usually make allegations of child abuse, but simply to remind clinicians that parents litigating in a custody battle may have other motivations (intentional or otherwise) for alleging child abuse on the part of the other parent. For example, one parent may attempt to use triangulation to place the therapist in the "abuse validator" role (Ellis, 2006).

Because mandated reporting laws vary from state to state, it may be helpful to use federal reporting standards as a reference point. In 1974, Congress enacted Public Law (PL) 93-247, known as the National Child Abuse Prevention and Treatment Act (CAPTA; 1974), 42 U.S.C. § 5101, *et seq.* This federal law provided model legislation for states to pass mandatory child abuse reporting laws. Enacted in 1974 as Public Law 93-247, CAPTA was amended in 2003 as PL 108-36, known as the Keeping Children and Families Safe Act, 42 U.S.C. § 5101 *et seq.* CAPTA provides a general definition of child abuse:

> Physical or mental injury, sexual abuse or exploitation, negligent treatment, or maltreatment of a child under the age of eighteen or the age specified by the child protection law of the state in question, by a person who is responsible for the child's welfare, under circumstances which indicate that the child's health or welfare is harmed or threatened thereby.

In addition, CAPTA sets forth a minimum definition of child abuse that includes any recent act or failure to act on the part of a parent or caretaker which results in death, serious physical or emotional harm, sexual abuse or exploitation; or an act or failure to act which presents an imminent risk of serious harm. CAPTA mandates "minimum definitions" for child abuse and sexual abuse.

Child abuse or neglect is any recent act or failure to act:

- Resulting in imminent risk of serious harm, death, serious physical or emotional harm, sexual abuse, or exploitation
- Of a child (usually a person under the age of 18, but a younger age may be specified in cases not involving sexual abuse)
- By a parent or caretaker who is responsible for the child's welfare

Sexual abuse is defined as the following:

- Employment, use, persuasion, inducement, enticement, or coercion of any child to engage in, or assist any other person to engage in, any sexually explicit conduct or any simulation of such conduct for the purpose of producing any visual depiction of such conduct; or
- Rape, and in cases of caretaker or inter-familial relationships, statutory rape, molestation, prostitution, or other form of sexual exploitation of children, or incest with children

One important question relates to the threshold required for the presence of *reportable* child abuse. Although child abuse is defined differently in different states, all states are required by CAPTA to have provisions for the protection of children. All 50 states have some form of a mandatory child abuse and neglect reporting law in order to qualify for federal funding under CAPTA. The specific wording of state laws is important to understand because "statutory wording is one of the variables that actually determines whether or not a mandated reporter will report suspected abuse (Kalichman, 1993, p. 63; Kalichman & Craig, 1991). For these reasons, it is sometimes helpful to read fine print of specific state child abuse reporting laws. For example, for Florida mandated reporters, Chapters 39.201 (1[a]) of the Florida Statutes states, "Any person who knows, or has reasonable cause to suspect, that a child is abused, abandoned, or neglected by a parent, legal custodian, caregiver, or other person responsible for the child's welfare" (Reporting Child Abuse, 2005). Chapter 415.101 of the Florida Statutes requires similar mandated reports to be made in cases involving suspected abuse of vulnerable adults.

For Georgia mandated reporters, the Child Abuse Reporting laws are contained in the Chapter 19-7-5 and Chapter 49-5-40 or the Official Code of Georgia Annotated (O.C.G.A.). According to the Georgia Code, the threshold for reporting child abuse is a "reasonable cause to believe" that a child under age 18 has been abused by a parent or a caretaker. "Reasonable cause" means that a reasonable person has a suspicion based on circumstances sufficiently strong to warrant a belief that abuse could have occurred (McGarrah, 2001). When, where, and how do you have to report suspected abuse? Georgia law states that the report must be made "immediately, but in no case later than 24 hours from the time there is reasonable cause to believe a child has been abused, by telephone or otherwise and followed by a report in writing, if requested, to a child welfare agency providing protective services, as designated by the Department of Human Resources, or, in the absence of such agency, to an appropriate police authority or district attorney" (O.C.G.A. 19-7-5[e], effective July 1, 2006). Is spanking considered child abuse? Under Georgia law, "physical forms of discipline may be used as long as there is no physical injury to the child." What about "emotional abuse"? Georgia law defines reportable abuse as physical injury other than accidental means; neglect and exploitation; and sexual abuse or exploitation. "Emotional abuse" is not statutorily defined in some states (including Georgia law), but for reporting purposes emotional abuse may be subsumed under the broad definition of neglect, and emotional abuse is sometimes associated with other forms of abuse. Other states do contain specific statutory definitions and requirements regarding emotional abuse. In Tennessee, for example, emotional abuse includes verbal assaults, ignoring and indifference, or constant family conflict.

As mentioned previously, a parent's allegations of child abuse by the other parent are sometimes used as a strategic form of triangulation designed to place the therapist in the "abuse validator" role. The ultimate goal of such a strategy is to get the therapist to testify against the other parent during a custody battle. Ellis (2006) provides the following example of how an unwitting therapist can slide down the slippery slope into the abuse validator pitfall:

> A mother brings a child or children to see you "for counseling." The parents have just separated and the mother has filed for divorce, alleging the children have been "abused" by the father or alleging that the father is somehow mentally unstable or neglectful. She has asked that you not involve the father in their treatment as it would be "too traumatic" for the children. The

mother is clear that she is not asking you to be involved in a
court proceeding but simply to provide treatment. After you have
seen this same parent and children a few times, this parent asks
you to write a letter or a report stating that the children are too
traumatized to see their father. (p. 12)

Given the preceding scenario, what do you do? Do you comply with
the mother's request? Do you write a letter based on such limited and
biased information? Do you call the father despite the mother's request?
According to Ellis (2006), in any treatment scenario with children, it is
important to involve both parents, even if it is by phone to the parent in
another state. A parent's request for the therapist to not contact the other
parent should be viewed by the therapist as a strategic maneuver to procure
the therapist's opinion in a custody proceeding. The ethically conscientious
therapist will make it clear from the outset that he or she would like to
interview the other parent to obtain history and remain in touch with that
parent to provide feedback. In other words, make it clear that you cannot
provide treatment to the child while totally excluding the other parent.
Ellis indicates that some clinicians ask the parent who is requiring
treatment while in the middle of a divorce proceeding to sign an agreement
stating he or she will not subpoena the clinician to consult with his or her
attorney, submit a letter to the court, or attend a judicial hearing. Of course,
such an agreement does not eliminate the possibility that the parent might
try to manipulate the situation, but such an agreement does help manage
the client's expectations from the outset.

Duty to Protect

If you suspect that one of your clients might be dangerous to someone,
do you have a duty to warn anyone? What if your client discloses to you
a specific threat against a readily identifiable target victim? What if your
client specifies no one at all? What if you have no ability to control your
client after he or she angrily walks out of your office? These questions
represent some of the most complex and troublesome ethical dilemmas
that confront mental health professionals. Whereas the reporting of child
abuse is mandated by law in all 50 states, the so-called duty to warn is
more complex because the decision is usually based on the discretion
and professional judgment of the therapist. According to APA Ethical
Standard 4.05(b) (Disclosures), psychologists may disclose confidential
information to "protect the client/patient, psychologist, or others from
harm" (p. 1066). The APA standard is permissive ("may disclose") rather

Chapter 5 – Consulting With Colleagues: Don't Worry Alone   149

than mandatory ("shall disclose"). Although the APA standard *permits* disclosure to protect others, it does not *require* disclosures to warn others. In other words, what is often perceived as a duty to *warn* others is in reality a duty to *protect* others. Similarly for counselors, ACA Section B.2.a. states, "The general requirement that counselors keep information confidential does not apply when disclosure is required to protect clients or identified others from serious and foreseeable harm or when legal requirements demand that confidential information must be revealed" (p. 7). Although both sets of standards permit disclosure to *protect* others, neither set of standards requires disclosures to *warn* others. In other words, the so-called duty to warn others is in reality a duty to protect others.

Disclosure laws, which vary from state to state, generally come in two forms. *Statutory laws* are laws that are legislated by state general assemblies and signed into law by the Governor, whereas *case laws* are legal precedents that are adjudicated by appellate courts and signed by Judges. In Georgia, there is no mandatory statutory duty to warn an identfiable third party of harm, nor is there any statutory immunity from legal liability for psychologists who make such warnings. Because Georgia is one of many states that has codified the APA (2002) Ethics Code into its licensing board rules, there does exist a permissive standard allowing such discretionary disclosure although this licensing board rule neither mandates such disclosure nor does it provide immunity or protection for psychologists making such disclosures. For example, under Section 4.05 (Disclosures) of Chapter 510-4-.02 (Code of Ethics) of the Georgia Rules of the State Board of Examiners of Psychologists (2004), there is a discretionary allowance for a licensed psychologist to disclose confidential information in order to "protect the client/patient, psychologist, or others from harm" (p. 6). However, this licensing board standard does not have the full force of *statutory law* but rather represents an *administrative rule* under which licensed psychologists practice.

Georgia also has a legal precedent that establishes a duty to protect third parties as defined by case law (*Bradley Center, Inc. v. Wessner, et al.*, 1982). In *Bradley v. Wessner*, the court determined a failure to exercise control over a potentially violent inpatient who made a clear threat toward a readily identifiable intended victim. In affirming the appellate decision below, the Georgia Supreme Court held that the Court of Appeals properly identified the legal duty in this case:

> Where the course of treatment of a mental patient involves an exercise of "control" over him by a physician who knows or should know that the patient is likely to cause bodily harm to others, an independent duty arises from that relationship and falls

upon the physician to exercise that control with such reasonable care as to prevent harm to others at the hands of the patient. (*Bradley Center v. Wessner*, 161 Ga. App. 576, *supra*, at 581, 1982)

Because the Bradley case specifically involved a hospitalized patient over whom some control could have been exercised by the psychiatric hospital, the case may have limited applicability in outpatient settings where less control can be exercised by the individual practitioner. Furthermore, the case did not involve any duty to warn, but instead involved the negligent release of a dangerous patient. In this respect, the case was similar to other cases involving failure to control a dangerous patient (e.g., *Jablonski v. United States*, 1983).

Although Georgia case law has established a legal precedent for a duty to *protect*, there is no statutory duty to *warn*, nor is there any statutory immunity for a psychologist making such a warning to a third party. In other words, although there is a legally established duty to protect a readily identifiable intended victim, there is no statutory duty to warn the victim nor is there any statutory protection from legal liability for mental health professionals who make such warnings. Although the case was never appealed and therefore never established as legal precedent, in *Garner v. Stone* (1999), a six-person jury in a DeKalb County, Georgia, state court found in favor of a former police officer with Gwinnett County, Georgia, who sued a psychologist for violating the physician-patient privilege after the psychologist made a warning call to an identifiable third party. According to the court records, during a fitness-for-duty interview conducted by a consulting psychologist on August 30, 1996, the police officer disclosed that he had had a vision of killing his captain and thoughts about killing 8 to 10 others including the police chief and a county commissioner. The psychologist took the matter seriously and eventually reported the conversation to the police officer's superiors. Attorneys for the plaintiff argued that their client's conversation with the psychologist was absolutely privileged and that state law provided no exception to the privilege. Attorneys for the defendant psychologist argued that psychologists have a duty to warn third parties if a patient is likely to cause bodily harm. The defense argued that Georgia courts have imposed a duty on mental health professionals to use reasonable care to prevent harm to third parties from a dangerous patient, but the courts have not specifically defined a duty to warn third parties in such situations. It is noteworthy that the psychologist's affidavit indicated that he "did not believe the threats to be imminent but considered them to be very serious."

Interestingly, the trial judge's charge to the jury included discussion of the discretionary allowance under the Georgia Code of Conduct, which permits psychologist disclosure to prevent harm to the patient or others, as well as discussion of the California *Tarasoff* ruling, which is legally binding only in the state of California.

The *Tarasoff* case is so central to the understanding of the duty to protect that it deserves some discussion. *Tarasoff v. Board of Regents of the University of California* (1976) was the California Supreme Court ruling that was the result of a series of appeals in the civil suit filed by the family of Tatiana (Tanya) Tarasoff, a University of California at Berkeley student who was killed by Prosenjit Poddar on October 27, 1969. What has become known as the *Tarasoff* decision has been the source of almost endless confusion, including the fact that there was a criminal court decision, a trial court civil decision, an appellate decision, and a California Supreme Court ruling. Another source of confusion about *Tarasoff* is that the California Supreme Court issued two separate rulings in the case, the first of which was a "duty-to-warn" decision and the second of which was a "duty-to-protect" decision (sometimes referred to as Tarasoff II) that nullified and replaced the first decision. The facts of the case indicate that immediately after Tanya was fatally stabbed with a kitchen knife, Poddar returned to Tanya's house and he called the police. Poddar's defense lawyers argued "diminished capacity" and produced one psychologist and three psychiatrists who testified that he was paranoid schizophrenic and could not have harbored "malice with forethought." The prosecution's court-appointed psychiatrist argued that Poddar was only schizoid and therefore a verdict of first- or second-degree murder was appropriate. After a seemingly straightforward conviction based on a 17-day trial, a jury of Superior Court of Alameda County found Poddar guilty and he was convicted of second-degree murder. However, the criminal trial court's decision was overturned on appeal on February 7, 1974. The verdict was reversed because the judge had erred in his instructions to the jury by failing to give adequate instructions concerning the defense of "diminished capacity" (*People v. Poddar*, 1974). Poddar was convicted of voluntary manslaughter, confined to the Vacaville medical facility in California, and later released whereupon he returned to his homeland of India. The last information on Poddar was reportedly a letter in which he stated that he "has returned to India, and by his own account is now happily married" (Stone, 1976, p. 358).

At the same time the criminal trial was taking place, the Tarasoff family filed a civil suit against the Board of Regents of the University of California and its employees. The malpractice suit claimed failure to commit Poddar and failure to warn Tanya of danger. In 1974, the lower court dismissed the civil action against the University, finding that there was no cause of action because the University owed no duty of care to Tatiana because she was not their patient but rather just a third party. Tatiana's parents appealed the lower court ruling to the California Supreme Court, which reversed the decision of the lower court and allowed Tatiana's parents to maintain their cause of action against the University for the failure to warn. The case was remanded back to the district court for a retrial. The *Tarasoff* opinion did not decide whether the University had been negligent. Instead, the court simply held that the Plaintiff had stated a cause of action that, if proved at trial, would have entitled Tatiana's parents to relief from damages. Theoretically, on remand to the lower court, the trier of fact would have had to decide whether the University's failure to notify the victim or her family did in fact constitute a breach of the duty to the third-party victim. On the other hand, it is possible that the trial court could have found that by notifying the police, the University had exercised due care and was not negligent. The outcome remains forever unknown because the civil case was settled by the parties out of court prior to a retrial.

In the *Tarasoff* civil suit, both the original trial court and the initial appeal court held for the defendants. It was only when the case reached the California Supreme Court that the plaintiff's arguments were finally upheld. On December 24, 1974, the California Supreme Court issued its first *Tarasoff* ruling:

> When a doctor or a psychotherapist, in the exercise of his professional skill and knowledge, determines, or should determine, that a warning is essential to avert danger arising from the medical or psychological condition of his patient, he incurs a legal obligation to give that warning.

The California Supreme Court decision caused such an upheaval, mainly among psychiatrists and psychologists, that the court agreed to take the rare step of rehearing the case. When they agreed to do this, the December 24, 1974 decision became null and void, as if it had never existed. On July 1, 1976, the Supreme Court rendered what was to be the definitive *Tarasoff* ruling, which differed in significant ways from the December 24, 1974 decision. In its 1976 decision, the court held the following:

> We shall explain that defendant therapists cannot escape liability merely because Tatiana herself was not their patient. When a

therapist determines, or pursuant to the standards of his profession should determine, that his patient presents a serious danger of violence to another, he incurs an obligation to use reasonable care to protect the intended victim against such danger. The discharge of this duty may require the therapist to take one or more of various steps, depending upon the nature of the case. Thus it may call for him to warn the intended victim or others likely to apprise the victim of the danger, to notify the police, or to take whatever other steps are reasonably necessary under the circumstances.

The California Supreme Court's original 1974 "duty-to-warn" opinion was later nullified and modified in 1976 to a "duty-to-protect" opinion. The so-called *Tarasoff* threshold is reached when there is a clear threat against an identifiable potential victim. In 1985, the California legislature enacted Section 43.92 of the California Civil Code, which limits the liability of psychotherapists when a patient makes a serious threat of violence. When there is a duty to warn and protect under the limited circumstances specified in the California law, "the duty shall be discharged by the psychotherapist making reasonable efforts to communicate the threat to the victim or victims and to a law enforcement agency" (California Civil Code, Section 43.92, 1985). Several state psychological associations have considered the pros and cons of introducing immunity legislation to protect psychologists who make so-called *Tarasoff* warnings.* Since

---

*Immunity statutes typically include language that (a) defines the psychotherapist's duty and limits of liability in cases involving a serious threat of physical violence against a reasonably identifiable victim or victims, (b) establishes statutory immunity from liability for psychotherapists who in good faith comply with this requirement, and (c) identifies the licensed practitioners to whom this requirement would apply. Model legislation proposed by Remar (2000) and discussed by Doverspike (2007) includes the following elements:

(1) A psychotherapist shall not be held liable in any civil action for failing to warn of and/or protect from a patient's threatened violent behavior or for failing to predict and warn of and/or protect from a patient's violent behavior except in those instances where the patient has communicated to the therapist a serious threat of physical violence against a reasonably identifiable victim or victims.

(2) If a duty arises under subsection (1) of this Code Section, the duty shall be discharged by the psychotherapist making reasonable efforts to communicate the threat to the victim or victims or to a law enforcement agency. Notwithstanding that the patient's communication to the psychotherapist is otherwise made privileged or confidential by law, a psychotherapist who in good faith communicates the threat to the victim or victims or to a law enforcement agency shall be immune from liability for said communication.

(3) As used in this Code Section, the term "psychotherapist" shall be defined as a psychiatrist, licensed psychologist, licensed clinical social worker, clinical nurse specialist in psychiatric/mental health, licensed marriage and family therapist, or licensed professional counselor.

California enacted the first limited liability statute in 1985, 23 states have passed similar legislation applicable to mental health professionals, and a significant number of state courts have reviewed *Tarasoff*-type claims under these statutes. A review of these cases indicates that even in states that have *Tarasoff* statutes, "clinicians must continue to rely on their clinical and ethical judgment, rather than statutory guidance, when considering potential protective disclosures or future drafts of protective disclosure statutes" (Kachigian & Felthous, 2004, p. 263).

Legal standards related to duty-to-protect others continue to evolve in case law. For example, in *Ewing v. Goldstein* (2004), a California appeals court expanded the *Tarasoff* duty for all California psychotherapists, who must heed credible warnings about a client's threatened violence from the client's immediate family members, as well as threatening statements from the clients themselves. In *Ewing v. Goldstein*, a former police officer who was undergoing psychotherapy carried out a homicidal threat against a man who was newly involved in a relationship with the former police officer's ex-girlfriend. The appellate court noted that when a communication of the serious threat of physical violence is received by a therapist *from a member of the patient's immediate family* (in this case, the patient's father) and is shared for the purpose of facilitating and furthering the patient's treatment, the fact that the family member is not technically a "patient" does not defeat or nullify the psychotherapist-patient privilege.

Notwithstanding the limited liability statutes that exist in some states such as California, there has been little initiative in other states to support a sustained drive for such legislative changes. There are also some inherent risks in introducing immunity legislation, which conceivably could erode the protective privilege that currently exists in psychologist-patient communications. The protective privilege in all 50 states has been considered so important that it has been affirmed by the United States Supreme Court (*Jaffee v. Redmond*, 1996). However, it is interesting to note that the Supreme Court ruling contains a footnote allowing for an exception to privilege "if a serious threat of harm to the patient or to others can be averted only by means of a disclosure by the therapist" (p. 18). Citing from *Jaffee v. Redmond*, Footnote 19 reads as follows:

> Although it would be premature to speculate about most future developments in the federal psychotherapist privilege, we do not doubt that there are situations in which the privilege must give way, for example, if a serious threat of harm to the patient or to

others can be averted only by means of a disclosure by the therapist. (p. 18)

How accurately must a therapist predict violence? According to Stromberg, Schneider, and Joondeph (1993), a therapist is required to predict violence at least as well as is customary among his or her colleagues, although this requirement confuses the issue of diagnosis (for which there is an accepted professional standard) and prediction (for which there may not be an accepted standard). Mental health professionals do not have a duty to accurately *predict* violence, but they do have a duty to adequately *assess* potential for violence. Adequate treatment is based on adequate assessment, and adequate assessment is based on a multiplicity of factors. These factors include obtaining a detailed patient history with a corroborative parallel history; conducting a careful review of current and prior treatment records; asking direct questions about the patient's violent ideation, intentions, actions, or plans; directly questioning the patient about access to weapons or other potentially lethal means; considering the "weapons effect" (Berkowitz, 1974); considering the "base rate" effect (Monahan, 1981); and so forth. The *weapons effect* refers to the phenomena first identified by Berkowitz and LePage (1967), in which the mere presence of a weapon may instigate the expression of aggression even if the weapon is not actually used to express aggression. Berkowitz made the argument explicit and summarized his observations with a slogan that has often been repeated: "Guns not only permit violence, they can stimulate it as well. The finger pulls the trigger, but the trigger may also be pulling the finger" (Berkowitz, 1968, p. 22). The *base rate effect* refers to the difficulty predicting a behavior that occurs at a low frequency or base rate. Monahan (1981) states that the most common and most significant error made by clinicians in predicting violent behavior is the ignoring of information regarding the base rate of violence in the general population. The base rate dilemma is illustrated in the following example provided by Livermore, Malmquist, and Meehl (1968):

> Assume that one person out of a thousand will kill. Assume also that an exceptionally accurate test is created which differentiates with 95 percent effectiveness those who will kill from those who will not. If 100,000 people were tested, out of the 100 who would kill, 95 would be isolated. Unfortunately, out of the 99,900 who would not kill, 4,995 people would also be isolated as potential killers. (p. 84)

If you have a reasonable cause to believe that one of your clients presents an imminent risk of foreseeable danger to a readily identifiable third party, do you have a duty to warn? First, keep in mind that your primary duty is to your client, whereas you may have a secondary duty to protect others only in the specific circumstance in which your client presents a clear risk of serious danger to others. Second, consider some of the trends that have been shown to be significant in the literature (e.g., Monahan, 1981, 1993; VandeCreek & Knapp, 2001). These trends include *identifiability* of the victim, *specificity* and clarity of the threat, *foreseeability* of danger, and *ability* to contain and control the client (e.g., inpatient vs. outpatient). Third, consider that there are several reasonable actions that one can take in order to exercise the ethical duty-to-protect others without actually warning others (e.g., intensification of treatment, involuntary hospitalization, removing access to weapons, seeking the assistance of others, using secondary monitors, and so forth). In other words, the duty-to-protect others involves clinical management of the client, the last option of which may require the therapist to breach confidentiality by making a third-party warning. The warning call should be the last step, not the first step, in the management of the dangerous client.

In making the most ethically justifiable decision, carefully consider the benefits and risks of warning versus not warning the intended victim. For example, some possible *benefits* of warning the intended victim might include protecting the intended victim and thereby protecting the client from committing an action that could eventually harm the client (e.g., retaliatory aggression, prison sentence, and so forth). On the other hand, the benefits of not warning the intended victim might include protecting the client's privacy interests, maintaining confidentiality, building trust in the therapeutic relationship, and possibly reducing the risk of the intended victim engaging in preemptive violence toward the client. The *risks* of warning the intended victim might include violating the client's privacy, breaching confidentiality, eroding trust in the therapeutic relationship, and possibly precipitating the intended victim's preemptive strike against the client. Conversely, the risks of not warning the intended victim might include allowing harm to befall the intended victim and thereby creating harm to the client (e.g., arrest, prison sentence, living with feelings of guilt, and so forth). In considering overarching moral principles, Anders and Terrell (2006) state, "Though most therapists struggle with the idea of breaching confidentiality, one should keep in mind that the right to life of a third party supercedes the right of the client to keep trust, as the latter can be regained (albeit with difficulty) and the former cannot" (p. 15). A careful analysis of risks and benefits of various actions may help clarify the best course of action in a worst-case scenario.

If you do decide to make a third-party warning, consider enlisting the client's cooperation by obtaining his or her written authorization before making any warning call, which in some cases may be possible. If the client does not provide permission, then consider making the call in the presence of the client, which may help preserve trust in the therapeutic relationship and which may strengthen the client's reality-testing abilities and impulse control (Doverspike & Stone, 2000). Finally, know the statutory laws and legal precedents in your local jurisdiction. As with any legal question, always consult an attorney for legal advice before making a decision.

Termination of Noncompliant Client

Can you terminate psychotherapy with a client who threatens you? Can you terminate psychotherapy with an uncooperative client? Psychotherapists do not abandon clients, but this does not mean that you must accept every new referral or that you cannot terminate services with a current client. Perhaps some better questions would be the following: *When* can you terminate psychotherapy with a client? *How* can you terminate psychotherapy with a client? APA Ethical Standard 10.10 (Terminating Therapy) delineates when and how it is appropriate to terminate services with a client:

(a) Psychologists terminate therapy when it becomes reasonably clear that the client/patient no longer needs the service, is not likely to benefit, or is being harmed by continued service.
(b) Psychologists may terminate therapy when threatened or otherwise endangered by the client/patient or another person with whom the client/patient has a relationship. (p. 1073)

When can you terminate psychotherapy with a client? As stated above, the APA Ethics specifies four justifiable reasons for termination with a client. A professional relationship with a client may be ethically terminated when it becomes reasonably clear that (a) the client no longer needs the service, (b) the client is not likely to benefit from the service, (c) the client is being harmed by the service, or (d) the therapist is being threatened or otherwise endangered by the client or patient or another person with whom the client or patient has a relationship. It is not only ethically justifiable to terminate services with a noncompliant and threatening client, but it may be unethical to continue rendering service to a noncompliant or threatening client (Younggren, 2006).

How do you terminate therapy with a client? Regardless of the reason for termination, the process must be conducted in an ethical manner. APA Ethical Standard 10.10(c) (Terminating Therapy) states, "Except where precluded by the actions of clients/patients or third-party payors, prior to termination psychologists provide pretermination counseling and suggest alternative service providers as appropriate" (p. 1073). It is significant to note that the 1992 APA Ethics Code also contained an additional standard that may be helpful: Except where precluded by the client's conduct, the psychologist has a duty to "take other reasonable steps to facilitate transfer of responsibility to another provider if the client needs one immediately" (APA, 1992, p. 1606). Although this standard was removed from the 2002 APA Ethics Code in order to avoid creating an undue liability burden for psychologists, it is still a good standard of practice to follow because it encourages therapists to aspire to a higher standard of care.

Internet and
Electronic Media

Is it ethical to provide Internet therapy? Just as we are no longer a profession of generalists, we are also no longer a profession confined by geographic boundaries. The definition of e-therapy, which is sometimes called cybercounseling, ranges from simply using email to confirm or change appointments to the use of real-time chat lines and video-conferencing to conduct individual or group counseling. Notice that there is no use of the term *psychotherapy*, which implies direct contact with the client, although the ethical standards for psychotherapy do apply when providing e-therapy. The salient ethical dimensions of so-called e-therapy include informed consent, competence and credentials, exceptions to confidentiality, as well as privacy and security limits (G. Corey et al., 2007).

In contemporary science and medicine, technology often develops at a faster pace than emerging ethical and legal standards. In contemporary psychology, APA's development of ethical guidelines for e-therapy has been slower than the development of practice patterns based on the technology of Internet services. Many psychologists ask why the 2002 APA Ethics Code does not contain specific standards related to e-therapy, cybercounseling, or other Internet services. Implicit in all standards of Ethics Code is the assumption that ethical standards apply to *all* forms of services, whether provided in person, via electronic transmission, or otherwise. The phrase "electronic transmission" is further emphasized in five separate sections of the 2002 Ethics Code, which essentially defines the standards for services rendered via the Internet, telephone, or otherwise. Furthermore, the APA "Ethics Code applies to these activities across a variety of contexts, such as in person, postal, telephone, internet, and other electronic transmissions" (p. 1061). In other words, the ethical standards contain language designed for psychologists who provide services in person, via electronic media, or by other forms of communication. In addition, the APA Ethics Code does have specific requirements for those offering services electronically. APA (2002) Ethical Standard 4.02(c) (Discussing the Limits of Confidentiality), states: "Psychologists who offer services, products, or information via electronic transmission inform clients/patients of the risks to privacy and limits of confidentiality" (p. 1066).

In contrast to the lack of specificity in the APA Ethics Code, the American Counseling Association (ACA; 1999) provides specific guidelines for e-therapy and cybercounseling in its *Ethical Standards for Internet On-Line Counseling*. The Confidentiality section, which is the first section of the three-page document, contains standards related to (a) privacy information, including secured sites, nonsecured sites, general information, and limits of confidentiality; (b) informational notices, including security of the professional counselor's site, professional counselor identification, and client identification; (c) client waiver; (d) records of electronic communications; and (e) electronic transfer of client information. The second section of the document, titled Establishing the On-Line Counseling relationship, includes standards related to (a) the appropriateness of online counseling; (b) counseling plans, continuing coverage; (c) boundaries of competence; and (d) minor or incompetent clients. For example, the subsection governing boundaries of competence states, "Professional counselors provide on-line counseling services only in practice areas within their expertise and do not provide on-line counseling services to clients located in states in which professional counselors are not licensed" (p. 3). The third section of the document, titled Legal Considerations, contains two short paragraphs about legal liability insurance coverage, legal assistance, and technical assistance. With respect to some of the informed consent considerations that professional counselors exercise when using online counseling, the ACA (1999) document states the following:

> Professional counselors develop an appropriate intake procedure
> for potential clients to determine whether on-line counseling is

appropriate for the needs of the client. Professional counselors warn potential clients that on-line services may not be appropriate in certain situations and, to the extent possible, inform the client of specific limitations, potential risks, and/or potential benefits relevant to the client's anticipated use of on-line counseling services. Professional counselors ensure that clients are intellectually, emotionally, and physically capable of using the on-line counseling service, and of understanding the potential risks and/or limitations of such services. (p. 2)

A review of the literature reveals an emphasis on the importance of informed consent, particularly as it relates to limits of privacy and exceptions to confidentiality. As discussed by Maheu (2001), "many practitioners do not know how to completely remove patient files from their own computer hard drive, how to secure email transmissions to protect patient confidentiality, or how easily a patient can install a 'Trojan Horse' program into the practitioner's computer to download its contents onto a remote computer" (p. 23). In general, the following issues should also be considered when providing electronic services: the limited scope of e-therapy, the inherent risks of e-therapy, the lack of a personal presence that limits the therapeutic relationship, the lack of social and nonverbal cues that limits diagnostic assessment, and the likelihood that e-therapy may be inappropriate for certain high-risk groups (including those with so-called Internet Addiction Disorder).

Supervision Concerns

Do you have to "sign-off" on your supervisee's reports? Can you supervise more than one person? If you are asking these questions, you might not be ready to be a supervisor. For Georgia psychologists, Chapter Five of the Licensure Rules is defined as the Supplemental Code of Conduct, which is meant to address those areas not included in the APA Ethics Code (Chapter Four of the Licensure Rules). The dilemma described above is explained in two sections of this chapter, including Chapter 510-5-.02 (Definitions) and Chapter 510-5-.06([7][8] Delegation to and Supervision of Supervisees of Psychological Services).
According to E. Campbell and Webb (2005, p. 7),

these rules explain that licensed psychologists can delegate and supervise psychological services to three categories of individuals: (a) trainees (post-doctoral students, interns, and predoctoral students), (b) employees (as opposed to subcontractors) of the licensed psychologist, and (c) individuals who are also employed by the same employer (e.g. hospital, mental health center). If supervisees meet one of these criteria and licensed psychologists accept the supervisory role, then several requirements for supervision are outlined (510-5-.06[3][a][g]).

Psychologists should read these rules carefully in order to fully understand the context of supervision.

E. Campbell and Webb (2004, p. 7)* discuss some major points of the supervisory relationship and offer the following interpretation of postdoctoral supervision requirements:

1. The supervisee must be (a) qualified and (b) have the education and training to reasonably perform the expected services competently and ethically.
2. The supervisees must inform the client/patients of their supervisory roles and the right of the client/patients to confer with the licensed psychologist on any aspect of care.
3. The licensed psychologist (a) personally takes part in the intake process, (b) personally makes the diagnosis, and (c) personally approves and co-signs a treatment plan.
4. The licensed psychologist meets regularly with the supervisees concerning client/patients providing a minimum of one hour of supervision for every 20 hours of face-to-face client/patient contact by the supervisee.
5. Licensed psychologists may not supervise more than three supervisees without the authorization of the Licensing Board. Each level of training supervision has specific supervisory requirements that supercede this given number of supervisees. (p. 7)

Do you incur liability when you provide peer consultation to a colleague? Legal liability is incurred only when a professional has established a fiduciary duty or responsibility to a patient/client or supervisee. Supervision creates a fiduciary responsibility and a legal duty to a therapist's patient, whereas consultation does not create a fiduciary responsibility or legal duty to the consultee's patient (*Schrader v. Kohut*, 1999). Supervision and consultation are fundamentally different relationships with different duties, objectives, and responsibilities. It is

---

*Reprinted with permission.

consistent with well-established legal and professional standards to hold that a supervisor owes a duty of care to the patient. In contrast, a peer consultant does *not* bear a legal duty to the consulting therapist or to the consulting therapist's patient. As cited in the appellate ruling of *Schrader v. Kohut* (1999), there is no legal liability in the absence of a professional relationship:

> It is a well-settled principle of Georgia law that there can be no liability for malpractice in the absence of [a] physician-patient relationship . . . . In such cases, called classic medical malpractice actions, doctor-patient privity is essential because it is this relation which is a result of a consensual transaction that establishes the legal duty to conform to a standard of conduct. The relationship is considered consensual where the patient knowingly seeks the assistance of the physician and the physician knowingly accepts him as a patient. (p. 2)

A supervisor owes a legal duty to the supervisee as well as to the supervisee's patient/client. On the other hand, as established in *Schrader v. Kohut*, a peer consultant does *not* owe a legal duty to the peer consultee or to the consultee's patient. For example, if Therapist A consults with Therapist B about the clinical management of one of Therapist A's patients, then Therapist B does not incur liability with respect to Therapist A's patient. Furthermore, if Therapist B is providing peer consultation (not supervision) to Therapist A, then Therapist B does not incur liability to Therapist A. It is only when Therapist A is providing *supervision* to Therapist B that Therapist A incurs a legal liability to Therapist B as well as to Therapist B's patient.

Education
And Training

Can you require students in a graduate class in marital therapy to construct genograms of their families of origin? Can you require clinical psychology graduate students to participate in a discussion exercise in which they reveal information about their relationships with significant others, including intimate partners? Can you require graduate students in a human sexuality class to write term papers about their past sexual histories? These are typical of some of the calls that I receive from those involved in education and training. Interestingly, I receive very few calls from academic colleagues but a surprisingly large number of calls from their students.

In graduate training programs, there has been increasing attention given to the degree to which students and postdoctoral trainees should be asked to disclose personal information in classes and in supervision. The evolving trend has been to require disclosure of sensitive personal information from students only if such disclosure has been stated in the training objectives or if it is necessary to evaluate a student's personal problems. APA (2002) Standard 7.04 (Student Disclosure of Personal Information) addresses this concern as follows:

> Psychologists do not require students or supervisees to disclose personal information in course- or program-related activities, either orally or in writing, regarding sexual history, history of abuse and neglect, psychological treatment, and relationships with parents, peers, and spouses or significant others except if (1) the program or training facility has clearly identified this requirement in its admissions and program materials or (2) the information is necessary to evaluate or obtain assistance for students whose personal problems could reasonably be judged to be preventing them from performing their training- or professionally related activities in a competent manner or posing a threat to the students or others. (pp. 1068-1069)

Disclosures required of students and supervisees should always be related to educational objectives. For example, if a training program requires psychotherapy trainees to explore their countertransference projections or interpersonal interactions, which might involve discussion of relationships with significant others such as parents or peers, then this training objective should be clearly stated in the graduate student handbook. In other words, prevent an ethical problem from developing in the first place by managing student expectations in advance. It is called "informed consent." In addition, teachers and supervisors should avoid taking on therapeutic roles with their students and supervisees.

Reporting
Ethical Violations

Should you file an ethics complaint against [fill in the name]? As mentioned previously, professional ethics committees usually perform two separate but related functions, including an *adjudicatory* role and an *advisory* role for their members. It is the advisory role that is relevant to the matter of consulting with colleagues, but it is the adjudicatory role for which I receive calls from consultations from colleagues who are interested in filing a complaint about a perceived ethical violation of another colleague. The typical allegation often comes in the form of the question, "I think it is unethical for so-and-so to [fill in the blank]. What do *you* think?" Whenever I hear this question, I first want to know which Ethical Standard, specifically, the inquiring colleague believes has been violated. Next, I wonder what motivates the inquiring colleague to be more concerned with the ethical behavior of others rather than with the ethical behavior of himself or herself.

APA (2002) Ethical Standard 1.04 (Informal Resolution of Ethical Violations) states, "When psychologists believe that there may have been an ethical violation by another psychologist, they attempt to resolve the issue by bringing it to the attention of that individual, if an informal resolution appears appropriate and the intervention does not violate any confidentiality rights that may be involved" (p. 1063). Similarly for counselors, Section H.2.b. of the ACA Code of Ethics (2005) states, "When counselors have reason to believe that another counselor is violating or has violated an ethical standard, they attempt first to resolve the issue informally with the other counselor if feasible, provided such action does not violate confidentiality rights that may be involved" (p. 19). In other words, the first step is not to file a complaint but rather to attempt to bring the matter to the attention of the offending colleague.

Although it is generally advisable to bring an ethical matter to the attention of the colleague who is suspected of unethical behavior, there are some exceptions to this general rule. If an ethical violation has substantially harmed a client or others and if an informal resolution of the matter is not appropriate, then other actions may be appropriate. Under APA (2002) Ethical Standard 1.05 (Reporting Ethical Violations), such actions may include "referral to state or national committees on professional ethics, to state licensing boards, or to the appropriate institutional authorities" (p. 1063). However, Ethical Standard 1.05 does not apply when the reporting of an apparent violation would violate the confidentiality rights of a client (e.g., your own psychotherapy client who specifically does not want the matter reported because to do so would violate his or her privacy rights). Pursuant to APA (2002) Ethical Standard 1.05, this standard also does not apply when a psychologist has been "retained to review the work of another psychologist whose professional conduct is in question" (p. 1063). For example, a forensic psychologist retained by a law firm as an expert witness would not necessarily be expected to report an opinion to a state licensing board, particularly if the psychologist was operating under an attorney-client privilege for the organizational client (i.e., the law firm).

Responding to
Ethical Violations in Organizations

Another common question involves how to respond to unethical or unacceptable circumstances that one observes in an organization in which one is working. Ethical decisions in community agencies, psychiatric hospitals, and other organizational settings are more complex and more difficult to resolve than decisions pertaining to individual counseling. The first step in responding to an unacceptable circumstance is to identify the problem and recognize the need for action. According to Homan (2004), once an agency problem has been identified in an organization or institution, there are four basic options from which to choose:

- You can change your perception by identifying the situation as acceptable.
- You can recognize the situation as unacceptable and then decide to adjust to the situation.
- You can leave the situation, either by emotionally withdrawing or by physically leaving.
- You can identify the situation as unacceptable and do what you can to change it.

In other words, you can accept the acceptable, accept the unacceptable, leave the situation, or change the situation. Each response corresponds to a psychological defense mechanism, such as *denial,* or not being aware of the unacceptable situation; *suppression*, consciously ignoring an unacceptable situation; *withdrawal*, leaving the situation, either emotionally (burnout) or physically (e.g., resigning); *rationalization*, such as reframing or accepting an abnormal situation as normal; or *self-assertion*, or doing something constructively as a response to the situation. Other defense mechanisms may include *acting out*, or taking impulsive actions rather than thinking or reflecting first; *passive-aggression*, indirectly or unassertively expressing aggression; *intellectualization*, such as using abstract thinking or making generalizations to control disturbing feelings; *humor*, laughing or joking about the situation; *sublimation*, channeling potentially maladaptive feelings or impulses into socially acceptable behavior; and so forth. Regardless of one's response to an unacceptable situation, each response has a consequence for the client, the therapist, and the organization. A consequential analysis, including use of the factorial matrix approach, can be helpful in evaluating the relative risks and benefits of various response options. Listed in alphabetical order, each one of these responses can be viewed as one of the following psychological defense mechanisms.

Acting out involves dealing with emotional conflict or external stressors by actions rather than by reflecting, processing, or verbalizing feelings appropriately. An example of acting out would be a social worker, with an excessively large caseload at a community service agency, who takes regular 3-hour lunches but informs his or her supervisor that he or she is making home visits to her home-bound clients during these hours.

Denial involves dealing with emotional conflict or external stressors through repression or by unconsciously refusing to acknowledge some painful aspect or subjective experience that would be apparent to others. Denial is the underlying defense mechanism exemplified in the expression "ignorance is bliss." An example of denial would be when colleagues in a pediatric group practice are not aware that one member of the practice is involved in the production of child pornography videos outside of the office setting.

Humor involves dealing with emotional conflict or external stressors by emphasizing the amusing or ironic aspects of the conflict or situation. An example would be a psychologist in a multidisciplinary private practice who pokes fun at the irony of the fact that the conflicts present in the practice mimic, in several ways, the conflicts present in many family systems.

Intellectualization involves dealing with emotional conflict or external stressors by the excessive use of abstract thinking or the making of generalizations to control or minimize disturbing feelings. An example would be a psychiatrist during a treatment team meeting who, when asked how he feels about the agency's new medical director, responds by explaining the theoretical model with which the medical director conceptualizes his treatment of patients.

Passive-aggression involves dealing with emotional conflict or external stressors by indirectly and unassertively expressing aggression toward others. Passive-aggression is sometimes seen in therapists who whine, procrastinate, show up late, don't return phone calls, or gossip about colleagues. An example would be a therapist who is always late turning in assignments, attending supervision meetings, and returning phone calls to his or her supervisor while complaining that his or her supervisor is never available.

Rationalization involves dealing with emotional conflict or external stressors by concealing the true motivations for one's own thoughts, actions, or feelings through the elaboration of reassuring or self-serving but incorrect explanations. An example would be a rural therapist who, after becoming aware that some of her clients in the agency are receiving prescriptions that are forged by one of the nonphysician therapists at the agency, explains to his or her clients that there is a shortage of physicians in rural areas.

Self-assertion involves dealing with emotional conflicts or external stressors by expressing one's feelings and thoughts directly in a way that is not coercive, aggressive, or manipulative. An example would be a practicum trainee who notices that the supervisor missed last week's supervisor session and the trainee politely but clearly reminds his or her supervisor that he or she is required by law to have a minimum of 1-hour face-to-face supervision each week.

Sublimation involves dealing with emotional conflict or external stressors by channeling potentially maladaptive feelings or impulses into socially acceptable behavior. An example would be a psychologist who, after becoming increasingly frustrated with the lack of clarity in a mandated reporting law, becomes a member of a political action committee that introduces legislation to rewrite the law with greater specificity.

Suppression involves dealing with emotional conflict or external stressors by intentionally avoiding thinking about disturbing problems, wishes, feelings, or experiences. Suppression may sometimes be reflected in a laissez-faire or "live and let live" philosophy. An example would be a therapist who decides not to get involved or say anything to a marriage counselor in his or her private practice who sells vitamins and herbs to the therapist's clients at the counseling center.

Withdrawal involves dealing with emotional conflict or external stressors by avoiding or leaving the stressor. Withdrawal can be emotional (burnout) or physical (leaving or resigning). Many enthusiastic mental health professionals who are in the midst of experiencing the newness of their careers have remarked to me that they "never want to become like" the tired, apathetic, and cynical staff members with whom they work. These enthusiasts are noticing burnout among their more senior colleagues. An example would be a therapist who, realizing that he or she has been emotionally burned out while working in a managed care setting, avoids interacting with colleagues, ignores phone messages, or turns in a letter of resignation.

Ethics and the Law

Do you know if there's a law on [fill in the blank]? If you need legal advice, call a lawyer—not a psychologist. Because the APA Ethical Standards are codified as licensing board rules in many states, it is sometimes difficult to separate ethical and legal standards. Consultations with a knowledgeable attorney can be helpful in differentiating legal and ethical standards. There are several ways that legal advice can be obtained. First, a practitioner can retain a private attorney. Secondly, a more cost-effective way of obtaining legal consultations is to use a professionally sponsored group legal services plan. For example, some state professional associations have Legal Service Plans that provide 1 or 2 hours per year for legal consultation. Finally, most professional liability insurance companies have risk-management hotlines that insured practitioners can call to obtain legal consultations.

If you want to save money on legal consultations, then read *The Psychologist's Legal Handbook* (Stromberg et al., 1988) before you call your lawyer. Become an educated consumer of legal services by learning to ask the right questions so that you use your legal consultation time effectively. Other excellent resources include some of the state specific reference books such as *Law & Mental Health Professionals: Georgia* (Remar & Hubert, 1996) and *Law & Mental Health Professionals: Florida* (Petrila & Otto, 2003), both of which contain a summary of state laws pertaining to mental health, psychology, and medicine. These reference books cost less than a 15-minute legal consultation. By reading the applicable section of the handbook before you consult with your attorney, you may be able to ask more specific questions and therefore use your legal consultation time more efficiently. In addition, practitioners can also obtain legal advice from the legal consultant of their professional liability insurance companies.

PSYCHOLOGICAL VERSUS LEGAL CONSULTATIONS

A respected colleague once told me that psychologists are on the verge of practicing law when they provide peer consultations regarding legal questions such as mandated reporting of suspected child abuse. I share my colleague's concern that many psychologists who request "ethics consultations" are in reality needing legal consultations. In my own experience, the majority of therapists who call to ask a "quick question" usually have a more complex legal question that is the crux of the matter. In fact, when conducting ethics workshops over the past several years, I try to avoid the "quick question" or the hallway consultation because in reality it is often the tip of the iceberg, under which lurks a more complex legal question complicated by clinical dynamics that would baffle even a master psychotherapist. Nevertheless, asking a psychotherapist for free legal advice is probably worse than asking an attorney for free psychotherapy.

In order to become licensed, most mental health professionals are required to demonstrate *knowledge* of applicable statutory and case law (knowledge competency) as well as *proficiency* in being able to integrate and apply such knowledge in practice (skill competencies). For example, Georgia psychologists are required to pass the Georgia Jurisprudence Examination (see Paragraph 2[c] of Chapter 510-2-.01 [Application by Examination]), covering "current laws, rules and regulations, and general provisions" (p. 1). The American Psychological Association (APA; 2002) Ethics Code explicitly states, "In the process of making decisions regarding their professional behavior, psychologists must consider this Ethics Code *in addition to applicable laws* [italics added] and psychology board regulations" (p. 1062). An underlying assumption in the APA code is that psychologists *understand* applicable laws and legal regulations. In fact, the word "law" is explicitly stated approximately 30 times throughout the APA Ethics Code, which itself is incorporated into psychology board rules and regulations in approximately 27 states—including Georgia.

To know one's ethical duty, a psychologist must also understand his or her legal duty (Behnke, 2005). A good place to start is by learning the laws and knowing how to integrate them into one's practice. In other words, know the code. Keep a desk reference, such as *The Psychologist's Legal Handbook* (Stromberg et al., 1988), *Law & Mental Health Professionals: Georgia* (Remar & Hubert, 1996), or *Law & Mental Health Professionals: Florida* (Petrila & Otto, 2003), and then do your homework. In other words, know which questions to ask when seeking a legal consultation—from an attorney. Get to know an attorney who has specialized knowledge and proficiency in mental health law. When consulting with a private attorney, be sure to discuss fees for legal services before you are "on the clock." Research relevant legal and ethical standards *before* making the call. Write down your questions in advance. Keep a written record of consultation. Mark your consultations with your attorney as Client-Attorney Privileged Communications.

If you don't wish to retain a private attorney, then call the risk-management service provided by your professional liability insurance company. Younggren (2005) advises practitioners to call at the first sign of a potential problem. If you wait until the problem has developed, it is much harder to limit the potential damage. In risk management, there is no such thing as a "stupid" question or unnecessary call. When you call your professional liability insurance company, your call will be answered by a member of the staff who will record some basic information and schedule an appointment for the risk-management consultant to call back and discuss your situation. When the consultant returns your call, be prepared to discuss the issues in some detail. Have your case files and other related documents readily available. In complex situations, the consultation may include a recommendation that you consult with an attorney, a clinical consultant, or both. Keep in mind that peer consultations are generally *not* considered legally privileged (Harris, 2004; Younggren, 2006). Your consultation is legally privileged only if it occurs with an attorney.

Regardless of whether you retain a private attorney or call your professional liability insurance company (or both), be sure to get an opinion specific to your state. Because there are significant differences in the statutory laws and legal precedents (case law) in different states, be sure to get a legal opinion based on the specific laws of the state in which you are practicing. Finally, remember that the most effective and least expensive form of liability insurance is good documentation (Schaffer, 1997). In plain English, keep good notes of your consultations, decisions, and actions.

In an ideal world, we are held accountable not for the accuracy of our predictions but in the reasonableness that has been taken in arriving at such predictions. Ethically responsible behavior is based on the assumption of a reasonable effort. Consulting with a colleague is an example of a reasonable effort. Consulting with a colleague is one of the best ways to achieve a reasonable standard of care. In my opinion, psychologists are not on the verge of practicing law when they discuss legal questions, but they are certainly on the verge of malpractice when they fail to provide a reasonable standard of care to their clients (Doverspike, 2006d).

SUMMARY OF CONSULTING
WITH COLLEAGUES

In summary, consult with a colleague when in doubt about a course of action. As Behnke (2005) succinctly states, "Don't worry alone." Every practitioner faces complex situations that require consideration beyond one's own best judgment. The wise practitioner knows when to consult with a peer. A good peer is someone who can help you see a different perspective, identify your ethical blind spots, and maximize your options for responding to the situation. An experienced colleague can often help distinguish the clinical dynamics from the ethical dilemmas of a case. An experienced colleague and an attorney can help you differentiate the ethical and legal standards of a case. Two heads are better than one, and a brief consultation is better than not consulting at all.

POINTS TO REMEMBER

- Consult with a colleague when in doubt about a course of action.
- Consulting with a colleague can help you see perspectives you have not considered.
- Consulting with a colleague can help you identify your ethical blind spots.
- Consulting with a colleague can help maximize your options for responding.
- Consulting with a colleague can help distinguish the clinical dynamics from the ethical dilemmas of a case.
- Consulting with a colleague and an attorney can help differentiate the ethical and legal standards of a case.
- Consulting with a colleague can help you feel more supported and less isolated.
- Facing ethical dilemmas in the present reduces the risk of complaints in the future.
- Ethics consultations are cheaper and take less time than depositions.
- Consultations help you aspire to excellence and practice risk management at the same time.
- Two heads are better than one, and a brief consultation is better than not consulting at all.

Chapter Six

Documentation and Record Keeping: Putting It in Writing

A psychologist who had been investigated by a state licensing board called me to express his frustration with the absence of due process during an investigation in which the investigator would not reveal the name of the complainant or the specific nature of the complaint. The psychologist lived in a state in which the licensing board was not required to inform the psychologist of the specific nature of the complaint. I suggested that the psychologist consult with an attorney, request from the state board the name of the person who had filed the complaint, and then obtain the client's permission to release the client's complete clinical record to the licensing board. Several months later, after the licensing board had closed the case as frivolous, I asked the psychologist how he had managed to defend himself against a complaint that was never revealed to him. He simply smiled and said, "I just gave them my notes, and I had *lots* of notes."

When psychologists ask for ethics advice, some of their most frequently asked questions relate to record keeping and documentation. These questions are very common, and their answers are usually relatively straightforward. APA (2002) Ethical Standard 6.01 (Documentation of Professional and Scientific Work and Maintenance of Records) states the following:

> Psychologists create, and to the extent the records are under their control, maintain, disseminate, store, retain, and dispose of records and data relating to their professional and scientific work in order to (1) facilitate provision of services later by them or other professionals, (2) allow for replication of research design

and analyses, (3) meet institutional requirements, (4) ensure accuracy of billing and payments, and (5) ensure compliance with law. (p. 1067)

In plain English, the APA standard means that your clinical records should be in compliance with the requirements of (a) Federal laws, such as the Health Insurance Portability and Accountability Act (HIPAA); (b) state laws, such as licensing board rules; (c) institutional requirements, such as agency or hospital regulations; and (d) any third-party payors, such as managed care companies with whom you have a contractual agreement.

RECORD RETENTION

How long should you keep psychological records? This question is a relatively common one to which there are several answers. Neither the APA (2002) Ethics Code nor the ACA (2005) Code of Ethics directly answers questions related to length of record retention or how much information should be kept in records. In order to answer questions related to record retention, one must consult other sources such as professional standards, federal regulations, and state laws.

Professional Standards

The APA (2007) *Record Keeping Guidelines* specify the following:

In the absence of a superceding requirement, psychologists may consider retaining full records until 7 years after the last date of service delivery for adults or until 3 years after a minor reaches the age of majority, whichever is later. In some circumstances, the psychologist may wish to keep records for a longer period, weighing the risks associated with obsolete or outdated information, or privacy loss, versus the potential benefits associated with preserving the records. (p. 10)

The above standard was foreshadowed by a footnote in the previous APA (1993) *Record Keeping Guidelines* which stated that, "if the specialty guidelines should be revised, a simple 7 year requirement for the retention of the complete record is preferred, which would be a more stringent requirement than any existing state statute" (p. 985). A review of the literature reveals at least one recommendation that the record be maintained for 10 years (Behnke et al., 1998). However, a 7-year retention period appears to be more consistent with the recommendations contained in ethics textbooks (e.g., G. Corey et al., 2003; Koocher & Keith-Spiegel, 1998). Compared to the 1993 APA guidelines, the most recent revision of the APA (2007) *Record Keeping Guidelines* proposes a more uniform standard: "In the absence of a superceding requirement, the psychologist may consider retaining full records for 7 years after the last date of service delivery for adults or for 7 years after a minor reaches the age of majority" (APA, 2007, p. 9).

Federal Regulations

Federal HIPAA regulations do not explicitly specify a period of retention for psychiatric, psychological, or mental health records (which are not differentiated in HIPAA). However, several sections of the regulations require that various forms of documentation (e.g., Accounting for Disclosures) be kept at least for the "previous six years." For example, in a section titled Patient's Rights and Psychologist's Duties, the model Georgia Explanation Form provided by the APA Practice Organization (2003) includes the following information under the heading of Documentation:

> A psychologist must document the titles of the persons or offices responsible for receiving and processing requests for access by patients and the designated record sets that are subject to access by patients. Psychologists must maintain a written or electronic record of any such documentation. Psychologists must retain this record for *six years* [italics added] from the date of its creation or the date when it was last in effect, whichever is later. (p. 10)

Explicit in the HIPAA regulations is the requirement that documentation of access and requests for records must continue to be maintained for as long as there are "requests for access by patients." Implicit in this requirement is the possibility that some records may need to be maintained indefinitely. If the HIPAA compliant provider receives a "request for access by patients" every 5 years, for example, then it is possible that the designated record set would have to be maintained indefinitely. In other words, it is within the realm of possibilities that the records would have to be maintained ad infinitum.

State Laws

Various state licensing laws differ in their requirements, and some state regulations do not even specify a length of record retention. In general, if the licensing board rules of a mental health profession do not address specific requirements such as record keeping, then practitioners licensed under those statutes are advised to consult the rules and regulations of other professions. The following discussion will focus on the regulations of one state with which I am familiar because I had the opportunity to review the draft version and make a recommendation before the regulations were adopted by the licensing board on November 23, 2004. My interpretation of these regulations is contained in three articles (Doverspike, 2005c, 2005d, 2006c), which provide the foundation for the following discussion. Because my analysis is based on the specific standards of the state regulations with which I am most familiar, practitioners in other states are advised to examine the specific requirements of their respective states. However, to the extent that the state regulation in question is based in part on the earlier APA (1993) guidelines, then the following discussion may have a broader applicability.

The current record retention rules contained in the Georgia Supplemental Code of Conduct (510-5-.04[2]), known as Maintenance and Retention of Records, are based on the APA (1987) model, although the additional 3-year retention period for a summary of the record is extended in the state regulations to an additional 8-year period. The Georgia standard not only requires a 7-year record retention period for the complete record, but it also requires an additional 8-year retention period for a summary of the record.

> (2) Psychologists are aware of relevant federal, state, and local laws and regulations governing records. Laws and regulations supercede requirement of these rules. In the absence of such laws and regulations, complete records are maintained for a minimum of seven years after the last date of service was rendered. A summary of the records are then maintained for an additional eight years before disposal. If the client is a minor, the record period is extended until three years after the age of majority. (p. 53)

Recommendations for
Adult Records

For adult records, a reasonable standard would be to keep the complete record for at least 7 years, and keep either the complete record or a summary of the record for a total of 15 years after the last date service was rendered. To provide greater access and to maintain a higher standard of care, HIPAA compliant providers should keep the complete record or a summary for at least 15 years after the last date of a request for access by the patient. To achieve the highest standard, keep the full record as long as is reasonably possible.

CHILD RECORDS

How long should you keep psychological records for children? Because requirements vary from state to state, I will give an example of the requirements of one state with which I am most familiar (Doverspike, 2005c), although these guidelines may have a broader applicability to other state regulations that are based on some combination of the APA (2007) model guidelines modified by the requirements of HIPAA. Chapter 510-5-.04 (Maintenance and Retention of Records) of the Georgia Supplemental Code of Conduct states in part, "Complete records are maintained for a minimum of seven years after the last date of service was rendered. A summary of the records are then maintained for an additional eight years before disposal. *If the client is a minor, the record period is extended until three years after the age of majority* [italics added]" (2004, p. 53). So what does this mean? Because the language is not explicit, it is subject to interpretation. For example, whereas the "age of majority" is not defined in this section of the Georgia Supplemental Code of Conduct, the consensus of most clinicians is to consider age 18 as the age of majority because this interpretation would be consistent with other sections of Georgia law (e.g., O.C.G.A. § 19-7-5). Nevertheless, this consideration is an *interpretation* of the rules rather than an explicit *specification* of the rules. A more complicated matter of interpretation relates to the intended meaning of the term "record period." Because various legal analysts and licensing board members have offered several possible interpretations, I will discuss two ends of the interpretive continuum as a preface to my own recommendation.

Conservative
Interpretation

Because the Georgia Supplemental Code of Conduct rules are subject to interpretation by the state board, it may be helpful to begin with a worst-case scenario interpretation of the term "record period." The most conservative record retention policy would be to keep the complete records until the former child client is 28 years old, and to keep some summary until the former client is 35 years old. Although this record retention period for minors may seem extreme, it is consistent with the more conservative interpretations that are often made by state licensing boards. For example, when I consulted a member of the Georgia licensing board on this matter (J. Currie, personal communication, January 23, 2004), it was explained to me that the record retention period for minor children *begins* at age 21, which is three years after the age of majority (18) in Georgia. Under this interpretation, the complete records of a minor would be retained for 7 years beyond age 21, and some summary of the records would be retained for a total of 15 years after age 21, which would mean that the former client would be 35 years of age at the time that the records could be disposed of. However, there are at least two problems with such an interpretation. First, such an interpretation operates under the assumption that the "record period" *begins* 3 years after the age of majority, whereas the actual statute states "the record period is *extended* [italics added] until three years after the age of majority" (Rules of the State Board of Examiners of Psychologists, Chapter 510-5-.04, 2004, p. 52). Secondly, this interpretation would also create inconsistent requirements for some records, because some child records would be required to be retained longer than some adult records. For example, under the conservative scenario described above, the complete records of a hypothetical 17-year-old client would have to be retained until the former client is 28 years old, yet the complete records of an 18-year-old client would have to be retained until the former client is only 25 years old.

Liberal
Interpretation

In contrast to the conservative interpretation described above, the most liberal interpretation of Chapter 510-5-.04(2) would yield an alternative record retention policy. A more liberal policy would be to keep the complete record of a minor child for 7 years after the last date of service or *until* the former child client is 21 years of age, *whichever period is longer.* In other words, the record period would be *extended* until 3 years after the age of majority, but in no case would the complete records be retained less than 7 years and in no case would a summary of the records be retained less than 15 years. However, keep in mind that this opinion is an *interpretation* of the standard, because such specificity of language does not actually exist in the statutory wording itself. One could argue that if the authors of the Georgia Code of Conduct had intended this meaning, then the standard would have been written this way in order to avoid any ambiguity. However, there are at least two problems with a liberal interpretation of this standard. First, because this interpretation creates a shorter record retention period, it does not afford the former client access to records as long as does the longer and more conservative record retention period stated in the previous section. Second, from a professional liability risk-management perspective, which takes into consideration the ambiguous wording of the Georgia standard, a shorter record retention period creates what is called a *period of uncertainty* during which it would be difficult for the psychologist to defend a claim that the record should have been maintained (J. Doverspike, personal communication, March 19, 2004).

It may be helpful to analyze a concrete example of the preceding liberal interpretation. If a hypothetical child client's last date of service occurred at age 5, then the conservative record retention policy would be to keep the complete record until the former child client is 28 years old (i.e., 7 years past age 21) and to keep a summary of the record until the former client is 36 years old (i.e., 15 years past age 21). In other words, the conservative policy in this case would require some type of record retention for up to 31 years. In contrast, the liberal record retention policy would be to keep the complete record until the former child client is 21 years old (i.e., at least 7 years, or 3 years past the age of majority, whichever is later) and to keep a summary of the record until the former client is 29 (i.e., at least 15 years, or 8 years past the age of majority, whichever is later). The longer and more conservative record retention period affords the client greater access to records while offering the service provider a decreased "period of uncertainty" should records be required in the future. From an aspirational ethical perspective, and also consistent with the intent of the federal HIPAA regulations, the psychologist's record retention policy should take into consideration client welfare in terms of the greatest degree of the client's access to records.

Recommendations
For Child Records

Consult with an attorney and adopt one of these policies depending on the nature of your practice, your degree of liability risk tolerance, and your ethical consideration of the welfare of your client. Client welfare should take into consideration the length of time and the degree to which you wish to afford former clients access to their records after services have been terminated. In summary, the conservative policy affords the benefits of greater client access and a reduced period of uncertainty weighed against the increased business costs of maintaining storage for a longer retention period. In contrast, the liberal policy affords the benefits of reduced costs of record storage for a shorter record period weighed against the increased costs of an increased period of uncertainty and decreased access to client records after services have been terminated. An optimal and reasonable balance of these costs and benefits can be derived from a policy in which the complete records of minor children are retained for a period of 15 years or until age 21, but in no case less than 15 years. Be advised that this policy is not specifically stated in the Georgia Code of Conduct, but rather is my own interpretation of the standard for the purpose of complying with the Georgia rules. My recommendation is to retain the complete former child client's record for a period of 15 years or until age 21, but in no case less than 15 years (Doverspike, 2005c). For example, the complete record of a 5-year-old former child client would be retained until the former client is 21 years old (i.e., the record period would be extended until 3 years past the age of majority), whereas the complete record for a 17-year-old former child client would be retained until the former client is 32 years old (i.e, 17 years plus 15 years).

PSYCHOTHERAPY NOTES

Do you have to keep psychotherapy notes? Professional standards and state laws require mental health professionals to maintain records, but such statutes do not specifically require mental health professionals to maintain psychotherapy notes. The HIPAA Privacy Rule allows clinicians to keep two sets of records, one of which would include the therapist's private psychotherapy notes that are segregated from the rest of the records, but the Privacy Rule does not mandate it. According to the interpretation of the APA Practice Organization (2002), the HIPAA statutory definition of Psychotherapy Notes consists of the following:

> Notes recorded (in any medium) by a healthcare provider who is a mental health professional documenting or analyzing the contents of conversation during a private counseling session or a group, joint, or family counseling session and that are separated from the rest of the individual's medical record. (p. 3)

According to the HIPAA Privacy Rule, "Psychotherapy notes are limited to only that information that is kept separate by the provider for his or her own purpose, and contain sensitive information relevant to no one other than the treating provider" (R. S. Smith, 2003, p. 6). In this respect, HIPAA Psychotherapy Notes are essentially the same as the type of notes that were traditionally known as process notes (*not* progress notes). *Process notes* may include not only facts, such as intimate details of a patient's personal life, but also details of dreams or fantasies, transference issues, free-associative material, and the therapist's subjective impressions of a client that are of interest only to the therapist. Rather than advising therapists to keep psychotherapy notes, legal analysts recommend that therapists keep progress notes (Harris, 2004; Stromberg et al., 1988; Younggren, 2005, 2006). *Progress notes* are factual, behavioral, and procedural in nature. They contain information on presenting problem, significant symptoms, psychiatric diagnosis, functional status, treatment plan, alternative treatments, therapist intervention, and client progress toward goals and objective. Progress notes are problem-oriented, behaviorally descriptive, and outcome-focused on treatment planning (Stromberg et al., 1988).

**Recommendations for
Psychotherapy Notes**

Don't keep psychotherapy *process* notes. Keep *progress* notes.

PROGRESS NOTES

How much detail should you put into your progress notes? This question should be answered within the context of the more general question: What has to be kept in records? As a point of historical reference,

APA (1987) *General Guidelines for Providers of Psychological Services* state that case notes minimally include dates and types of services as well as any "significant actions taken" (p. 717). The current APA *Record Keeping Guidelines* (2007) specify the following information that should be included in the client's file:

> Identifying information (e.g., name, client ID number); contact information (e.g., phone number, address, next of kin); fees and billing information; where appropriate, guardianship or conservatorship status; documentation of informed consent or assent for treatment (Ethics Code 3.10); documentation of waivers of confidentiality and authorization or consent for release of information (Ethics Code 4.05); documentation of any mandated disclosure of confidential information (e.g., report of child abuse, release secondary to a court order); presenting complaint, diagnosis, or basis for request for services; plan for services, updated as appropriate (e.g., treatment plan, supervision plan, intervention schedule, community interventions, consultation contracts); health and developmental history. (p. 6)

In addition to the preceding basic information that should be included in every client's record, the APA (2007) guidelines also specify the following information to be included in the record for each substantive contact with a client:

> Date of service and duration of session; types of services (e.g., consultation, assessment, treatment, training); nature of professional intervention or contact (e.g., treatment modalities, referral, letters, e-mail, phone contacts); formal or information assessment of client status. (p. 7)

Depending on the circumstances, the record may also include other specific information as delineated by the APA *Record Keeping Guidelines*:

> Client responses or reactions to professional interventions; current risk factors in relation to dangerousness to self or others; other treatment modalities employed such as medication or biofeedback treatment; emergency interventions (e.g., specially scheduled sessions, hospitalizations); plans for future interventions; information describing the qualitative aspects of the professional/

client interaction; prognosis; assessment or summary data (e.g., psychological testing, structured interviews, behavioral ratings, client behavior logs); consultations with or referrals to other professionals; case-related telephone, mail, and e-mail contacts; relevant cultural and sociopolitical factors. (p. 7)

State licensing laws usually contain information regarding the specific information that must be kept in records. For example, Chapter 510-5-.04(1) of the Georgia Supplemental Code of Conduct for psychologists specifies that records of psychological services include:

(1) identifying data; (2) dates of services; (3) types of services; (4) fees; (5) assessments; (6) treatment plan; (7) consultation; (8) summary reports and/or testing reports; (9) supporting data as may be required; and (10) any release of information obtained. (p. 53)

Because Chapter 510-5-.04 of the 2004 Georgia Supplemental Code of Conduct does not require the inclusion of some types of information (e.g., diagnosis) that were previously included in the "Maintenance and Retention of Records" section of the 1994 Supplemental Code of Conduct, it may be useful to review the types of information required for retention under the previous code. For licensed psychologists, Chapter 510-5-.03(7)(a) of the 1994 Georgia Code of Conduct specified that professional psychological records include:

(1) the presenting problem(s) or purpose or diagnosis; (2) the fee arrangement; (3) the date and substance of each billed contact or service; (4) any test results or other evaluative results obtained and any basic test data from which they were derived; (5) notation and results of formal consults with other providers; and (6) a copy of all tests or other evaluative reports prepared as part of the professional relationship. (p. 43)

Keep in mind that most managed care companies have published their own documentation guidelines that must be followed by providers who have signed contractual agreements. For example, Magellan Behavioral Health (1999) has published *Documentation Standards for Behavior Treatment Records*, which contains a provider checklist of 30 items that must be documented in the clinical record.

Recommendations for
Progress Notes

Combining the best of the old and the new versions of the Georgia Supplemental Code of Conduct, a progress note should minimally include identifying information, date of service, type of service, and documentation of any significant actions taken by the psychologist. A progress note may also include information such as session start and stop times, progress toward goals, specific interventions used to address objectives, and the patient's response to interventions. In addition to containing progress notes, the complete record of psychological services should minimally include (a) identifying data; (b) the presenting problem, reason for referral, purpose of sessions, and/or diagnosis; (c) types of services; (d) fees and financial arrangements; (e) assessments; (f) treatment plan; (g) summary reports, testing reports, test results, or other evaluative results obtained and any basic test data from which they were derived; (h) consultation, notation, and results of formal consults with other providers; (i) supporting data as may be required; (j) dates of service, including the date and substance of each billed contact or service; and (k) any release of information obtained.

RISK-MANAGED NOTES

How much time should you spend on writing notes, keeping records, and maintaining documentation? From a risk-management perspective, think of documentation as a business decision of how much time and energy are needed to justify your desired level of protection (Bennett et al., 1997; Harris, 2004; Younggren, 2002b, 2006). Psychologist/attorney Eric Harris often advises that progress notes should not only explain "what you did and why you did it" but also "what you didn't do and why you didn't do it" (e.g., Harris, 2004). Remember that good record keeping provides the first indication to a reviewer that your treatment meets minimum standards of care. In fact, case law supports the position that the quality of one's documentation may be taken as indicative of the quality of the services provided (*Donaldson v. O'Connor*, 1974; *White v. United States*, 1986; *Whitree v. State*, 1968).

In discussing the client record as a tool in risk management, Piazza and Yeager (1991) recommend that psychologists "not write anything in the client's records that you would not want a client's lawyer to read" (p. 344). Doverspike (1999b) suggests that you not only write your notes the way you would like to read them in court, but that you also "write your notes the way you would like someone *else* to read them in court" (p. 11). An even more paranoid documentation strategy is suggested by Gutheil (1980) who recommends, "In writing progress notes, trainees are urged to hallucinate on their shoulder the image of a hostile prosecuting attorney who might preside at the trial in which their records are subpoenaed" (p. 481).

Risk-management considerations aside, think of record keeping as an ethical decision of how much time and energy are needed to achieve your desired level of service to your *client*. Remember, "Reasonable clinicians protect themselves by protecting their patients" (Doverspike, 2004a, p. 210). Write your notes in a risk-managed way so that they can be read by your client's attorney in court, but also write them in a user-friendly way so that they can be read by your client in your office.

**Recommendation for
Risk-Managed Notes**

Write your progress notes in a user-friendly way so that they can be read by your client in your office, and write them in a risk-managed way so that they can be read by your client's attorney in court.

SUMMARY OF RECORDS

The Georgia Supplemental Code of Conduct (510-5-.04[2]) requires a 7-year record retention period for a complete psychological record, and it requires an additional 8-year retention period for a *summary* of the record.

> Psychologists are aware of relevant federal, state, and local laws and regulations governing records. Laws and regulations supercede requirement of these rules. In the absence of such laws and regulations, complete records are maintained for a minimum of seven years after the last date of service was rendered. A *summary of the records* [italics added] are [*sic*] then maintained for an additional eight years before disposal. If the client is a minor, the record period is extended until three years after the age of majority. (p. 53)

What is a "summary" of the record? Neither the 2004 Georgia Supplemental Code of Conduct nor the APA (2007) *Record Keeping Guidelines* defines what is meant by the term "summary of the record." In the absence of a clearly defined term, a prudent policy should take into consideration client welfare in terms of what kind of summary would provide the greatest benefit to the client. As a practical matter, it may be more cost-effective for most psychologists to simply retain the complete record, rather than spending time culling through each record in an attempt to retain only a summary.

For psychologists who have worked in institutional settings, it may be helpful to think of the summary as being similar to a hospital discharge summary. A *discharge summary* typically consists of a one- or two-page report that includes date of admission, reason for admission, preliminary diagnosis, brief history, course of treatment, discharge plan, final diagnosis, and prognosis. A summary of a psychological record would be different depending on the type of services rendered to the client. For example, in assessment and evaluation cases, a complete *psychological report* might be considered a sufficient summary, whereas in longer term cases a brief *closing summary* may be sufficient.

In psychotherapy cases, a more formal and comprehensive *closing summary* may be required, although the minimum requirement would be a termination note that provides a closing summary of the case. A closing summary typically includes a few of the elements that are required in a complete record, such as (a) identifying data; (b) presenting problem, reason for referral, purpose of sessions, and/or diagnosis (including admission and discharge diagnoses; (c) types of services rendered; (d) frequency of sessions; and (e) dates of services, including intake and termination dates. In addition to these elements and depending on the type of services provided to the client, a closing summary should also contain a termination note, documentation of treatment outcome, statement of prognosis, or documentation of the resolution of the presenting problem or the reason for referral.

Recommendations for
Summary of Records

For *assessment* records, consider retaining a summary of the record that includes (a) identifying data, (b) reason for referral, (c) type of evaluation, (d) dates of services, (e) assessment report, and (f) any recommendations. For *treatment* records, consider retaining a discharge or closing summary of the record including (a) identifying data, (b) presenting problem and/or diagnosis (including admission and discharge diagnoses), (c) types of services rendered, (d) dates of services, (e) termination note, and (f) documentation of treatment outcome or prognosis. In either case, clinicians are advised to consider that it may be more cost-effective to simply retain the complete record rather than spending time creating a summary of the record.

DISCLOSURE OF INFORMATION

What information needs to be included in an authorization for release of information? Clarifying the HIPAA requirements for an authorization form, the APA Practice Organization (2002) recommends that the following items be included in an authorization for disclosure of confidential information:

(1) a specific definition of the information to be used or disclosed, (2) to whom the information is going to be disclosed, (3) the purpose of the disclosure, (4) an expiration date, (5) the right to revoke, and (6) the right not to authorize the disclosure. (p. 6)

Some legal analysts (R. S. Smith, 2003, p. 8) have recommended that a HIPAA compliant authorization include the following items: (a) a specific description of the information to be used or disclosed, (b) name of the persons or class of people authorized to make the requested use or disclosure, (c) name of person(s) to whom information may be disclosed, (d) a description of each purpose of the requested use or disclosure, (e) an expiration date or event, (f) signature of the individual (or authorized representative), and (g) the date. It is significant that R. S. Smith includes the element of "a description of each purpose of the requested use or disclosure" because this information is necessary for the client to understand the implications or consequences of the disclosure. R. S. Smith (2003, p. 7) also states, "Authorization for psychotherapy notes cannot be combined with an authorization to release any other types of protected information nor can one be obtained for use in the future."

Although neither the HIPAA nor the APA standards make it an explicit requirement, authorized disclosure of confidential information should occur only after the client understands the implications of the disclosure.

As a point of historical reference, the APA (1987) *General Guidelines for Providers of Psychological Services* state, "Psychologists do not release confidential information, except with the written consent of the user involved, or his or her legal representative, guardian, or other holder of the privilege on behalf of the user, and only after the user has been *assisted to understand the implications of the release* [italics added]" (p. 21). In my opinion, it is unfortunate that the latest revisions of the APA ethical standards and the federal HIPAA requirements do not include this important requirement, because any competent client should always be assisted in understanding the implications of releasing confidential information. Nevertheless, a verbal discussion of the implications of releasing information should always accompany the written authorization for the release of information.

Recommendations for Disclosure of Information

Combining all of the above-mentioned elements, an authorization for the release of information should include (a) a specific description of the information to be used or disclosed, (b) name of the persons or class of people authorized to make the requested use or disclosure, (c) name of person(s) to whom information may be disclosed, (d) a description of each purpose of the requested use or disclosure, (e) an expiration date or event, (f) an explanation of the right not to authorize the disclosure, (g) an explanation of the right to revoke the authorization, (h) the signature of the individual (or authorized representative), and (i) the date.

CLIENT ACCESS

Do I have to give my patient a copy of my notes? A similar but more general question is: Does the patient always have a right to his or her records? The answers are "Yes and no." Although state laws and licensing board rules may differ from federal HIPAA regulations, most legal analysts and patient's rights advocates argue that competent adult patients generally have the right to access their records unless to do so would result in substantial harm to the patient. Where state laws provide patients with greater privacy protection and greater access to their records, state laws usually preempt HIPAA regulations for such purposes. In Georgia, for example, health care providers have traditionally relied upon the Official

Code of Georgia Annotated (O.C.G.A.) Chapter 31-33-2(a)(2), which specifies that, "Upon written request from the patient or a person authorized to have access to the patient's medical record under a health care power of attorney for such patient, the provider having custody and control of the patient's record shall furnish a complete and current copy of that record, in accordance with the provisions of this Code section." The only statutory exception to this requirement is in the case of patients for whom a disclosure may be harmful to the patient. Chapter 31-33-2(c) specifies that, "If the provider reasonably determines that disclosure of the record to the patient will be detrimental to the physical or mental health of the patient, the provider may refuse to furnish the record; however, upon such refusal, the patient's record shall be furnished to any other provider designated by the patient." However, deducing the applicable guideline for mental health providers is complicated by the fact that this statute does not even apply to psychologists and other mental health professionals. As O.C.G.A. Chapter 31-33-4 states, "The provisions of this chapter shall not apply to psychiatric, psychological, or other mental health records of a patient." Although the provisions of Chapter 31-33-4 do not apply to psychotherapists, the general rule is that patients (or their legal guardians) generally do have the right to access their records unless such access is determined to cause harm to the patient.

With respect to the federal standards, HIPAA generally favors the patient's access to his or her own medical records, although most legal analysts have a consensus of opinion that patients do not have access to the therapist's private "psychotherapy notes" that are maintained separate from the designated record set.

Recommendation
For Client Access

In order to comply with the spirit and intent of the APA Ethics Code as well as federal HIPAA standards, it is recommended that the psychologist provide the patient with access to his or her records unless such disclosure would be expected to result in "substantial harm" to the physical or mental health of the patient.

WRITTEN REPORTS

Do you have to give the client a written report? That depends on the contractual agreement made prior to services being rendered. These types of questions often arise in the case of third-party-referred Independent Consultative Examinations, which are sometimes referred to as Independent Medical Examinations (IMEs). APA (2002) Ethical Standard Section 9.10 (Explaining Assessment Results) specifies the following:

> Regardless of whether the scoring and interpretation are done by psychologists, by employees or assistants, or by automated or other outside services, psychologists take reasonable steps to ensure that explanations of results are given to the individual or designated representative unless the nature of the relationship precludes provision of an explanation of results (such as in some organizational consulting, preemployment or security screenings, and forensic evaluations), and this fact has been clearly explained to the person being assessed in advance. (p. 1072)

In some ways, the wording of APA Ethical Standard 2.09 (Explaining Assessment Results) of the 1992 code was clearer than the corresponding 2002 standard. APA Ethical Standard 2.09 (Explaining Assessment Results) of the 1992 Ethics Code reads as follows:

> Unless the nature of the relationship is clearly explained to the person being assessed in advance and precludes provision of an explanation of results (such as in some organizational consulting, preemployment or security screening, and forensic evaluations), psychologists ensure that an explanation of the results is provided using language that is reasonably understandable to the person assessed or to another legally authorized person on behalf of the client. (APA, 1992, p. 1604)

The APA (2002) standards do not state that a written psychological report must be prepared, but the standards do state that the patient is entitled to "explanations of the results" (p. 1072). If you do not plan to prepare a written report of results, make sure that you have clearly explained this to the patient in advance.

Recommendations
For Written Reports

Always prepare a written report of assessment results and inform the client in advance that there is a charge for the report. If the patient is not entitled to a written report of an evaluation that is requested by a third-party organizational client, make sure that you have obtained and documented the patient's understanding and agreement with this arrangement in advance. In other words, prevent an ethics problem by managing the client's expectations in advance.

SUMMARY OF DOCUMENTATION
AND RECORD KEEPING

From an aspirational ethical perspective, the quality of your documentation should reflect the quality of the services you provide. From a risk-management perspective, good documentation is the most effective and least expensive form of liability insurance. Write progress notes rather than process notes. In writing your notes, document what you did and why you did it, and document what you didn't do and why you didn't do it. Write your notes in a user-friendly way so they can be read by your client in your office. Write your notes in a risk-managed way so they can be read by your client's attorney in court. To achieve the highest standard of care in providing your client with the greatest access to his or her records, retain clinical records as long as is reasonably possible.

POINTS TO REMEMBER

- The quality of your documentation reflects the quality of the services you provide.
- Good documentation is the most effective and least expensive form of liability insurance.
- Write progress notes rather than process notes.
- Document what you did and why you did it.
- Document what you didn't do and why you didn't do it.
- Write your notes in a user-friendly way so that they can be read by your client in your office.
- Write your notes in a risk-managed way so they can be read by your client's attorney in court.
- Retain clinical records as long as is reasonably possible.

Chapter Seven

Responding Ethically to Complaints and Investigations: Turning Negatives Into Positives

Dear Reader:

The State Licensing Board would like to meet with you at an informal fact-finding inquiry before members of the Investigative Committee.

You should be aware that this proceeding is strictly voluntary, that your failure to appear will not be used against you at a formal hearing and will not be an admission to any wrongdoing. If you choose to appear, any statements you make or information gathered may be used against you at a formal hearing and be further used by the Board in determining what sanctions, if any, may be appropriate in your case. You may appear with or without an attorney. After an investigative interview is held, the Board may determine that an informal disposition of the case is appropriate or may decide that no action is warranted. If you decline to accept the Board's informal disposition, a formal hearing may be scheduled.

The Board would like to schedule an investigative interview at the Board office. Upon receipt of this letter, please immediately telephone and advise me as to whether you will attend, and I will then schedule a date and time for you.

Sincerely yours,

Board Member

Sooner or later, anyone could be faced with a situation in which one's best efforts must be explained in light of a complaint or investigation by a third party. In such situations, the best strategy is to have already followed some of the ideas that have been outlined in the previous chapters. These ideas include practicing within your area of competence, using an ongoing process of informed consent to create realistic client expectations in advance, managing boundaries appropriately, consulting with colleagues when in doubt about a course of action, and maintaining good record keeping and documentation.

RESPONDING TO THE
NOTICE OF INVESTIGATION

Known in some states as the "informal inquiry," some variation of the form letter on page 193 is often a practitioner's first notice that an ethics complaint has been filed by a former client. Acknowledging the certified letter as an "unpleasant experience" would be an understatement. An appropriate description of the experience would probably include a mixture of feelings such as anger and fear, panic and paranoia, or frustration and embarrassment. At a recent public gathering of psychologists, one colleague described the experience as being like a combination of a panic disorder and posttraumatic stress disorder. In many ways, the anxiety reaction is just like the litigation-induced posttraumatic stress disorders described in articles of *Medical Economics* magazine (referred to in Doverspike, 2005a). Amidst the flood of emotions that accompany this type of experience, there are some useful reminders that may be helpful to colleagues undergoing an ethics investigation.

THERE IS NO SUCH THING AS
A FRIVOLOUS COMPLAINT

A good starting point is to remember that there is no such thing as a frivolous complaint. Given the amount of time and the enormous emotional (and often financial) resources required to resolve formal complaints, it is important to take all client dissatisfactions seriously. A good working relationship may help guarantee that your client will report dissatisfactions directly to *you* rather than to someone else. In the event that your client does make a complaint directly to you, the best course of action would be to take the complaint seriously, discuss the client's concerns, obtain consultation with a peer, work toward a satisfactory resolution, and document your actions in writing (Doverspike, 1997c, 1999c). In the event that your client does make a complaint to a third party, such as a state ethics committee or licensing board, keep reading.

BE A COLLEAGUE,
NOT AN ADVERSARY

Before responding to the complaint inquiry, it may be helpful to remember that ethics committee members are your colleagues, not your adversaries. They are simply colleagues who have an interest in ethics education, who view their role as educative in nature, and who have been asked to volunteer their time by reviewing cases. Although licensing boards have a different role in protecting the public, board members are also your professional peers. Licensing board members are concerned with evaluating your behavior with respect to mandatory enforceable standards—not aspirational ethical ideals. When reviewing a therapist's response to an ethics complaint, there is probably nothing that an investigator likes more than to review a well-documented record that indicates that the practitioner in question provided a high standard of care. On the other hand, there is probably nothing that an investigator dislikes worse than to review a colleague's response of self-righteous indignation and arrogant rationalization of unethical behavior. Colleagues who are unjustly accused of wrongdoing are usually capable of rising to the occasion in a respectful and positive manner.

BE A BEHAVIORIST
WHEN EXPLAINING DETAILS

In formulating your response to a complaint letter, remember that your colleagues on the licensing board will not know anything about how you handled a case except for the information provided by you and the complainant. Because the complainant client has already filed a complaint, which is unlikely to portray your view of the situation, your main task is to explain your side of the story. Remember that your peer reviewers will not know your side of the story unless you provide the details. Regardless of your theoretical perspective, think like a behaviorist and explain what happened in terms of specific details, behaviors, events, and dates. It is important to focus on the details "with scrupulous attention" (Crawford,

1994, p. 92). If you kept good case notes, your record will be valuable in helping you recall specific details. If you did not keep good notes, remember Mark Twain's advice: "When in doubt, tell the truth."

EXPLAIN IN WRITING WHAT YOU DID AND WHY YOU DID IT

To use the rationale of Stromberg et al. (1988), explain what you did and why you did it, as well as what you didn't do and why you didn't do it. When making clinical and ethical decisions in difficult situations, a good clinical record should reflect a careful decision-making process. On an aspirational level, an ideal record would show (a) what your choice was expected to accomplish, (b) why you believed it would be effective, (c) any risks that might have been involved and why they were justified, (d) what alternative treatments were considered, (e) why they were rejected, and (f) what steps were taken to improve the effectiveness of your decision or chosen treatment (Soisson et al., 1987). When applying these guidelines to an ethics complaint investigation, remember that an ideal response should show a careful decision-making process or a coherent rationale for your actions.

BE SURE TO CITE THE STANDARDS

Because ethical decisions sometimes involve conflicting standards, be sure to cite the standards on which you based your decision. It is important to demonstrate to your peer reviewers that you understand the ethical standards and that you made a reasonable effort to follow those standards. For situations in which there are competing standards, it is important that you demonstrate how you resolved the conflict in a reasonable manner. Although it is important to know the mandatory or enforceable standards, it may be more important to demonstrate your concern for the aspirational standards. The merits of a complaint against you will be judged explicitly on the basis of your compliance with mandatory standards, although the virtues of your character will be implicitly evaluated on the basis of your concern with aspirational principles.

DO NOT
BLAME THE CLIENT

Individuals with severe characterological disturbance, particularly those with paranoid or borderline personality disorders, may be more likely to file complaints (Bennett et al., 1995, 1996, 1997; Harris, 2004; Harris & Remar, 1998; Younggren, 2006). However, don't think of the client's pathology as a defense of your behavior. Although you may feel like it, blaming the client is not a good response to a licensing board complaint. If the client is suffering from a severe characterological disorder, let the board draw their own conclusions based on the client's inappropriate actions and your appropriate responses. Your client's behavior may have been based on pathology, but your behavior should be based on principles. Because ethical decisions are based on principles, explain your actions and decisions in terms of *principles* and not *personalities*. Remember the adage, "Principles before personalities."

PUT PRINCIPLES
BEFORE PERSONALITIES

With the possible exception of the *cognizant* member of the licensing board, who knows the identity of the practitioner as well as the file number of the case, the other board members may know your case only by a file number. It is nothing personal; it is designed to be objective. For this reason, it is important that your response reflect your character. Licensing board investigations and ethics committee inquiries are generally concerned with the question of whether a practitioner's actions in a case fell below the enforceable ethical standards. In other words, the investigation is focused on the black-and-white standards that are codified in a formal document such as the APA (2002) Ethical Standards or the relevant state Code of Conduct. However, it is the virtue of your character that will fill in the gray areas of your response. Because board members may not know your good name and reputation in the community, let them know your character by the way that you respond to the complaint. Show that you are concerned with ethical principles and not with the personalities involved in adjudicating your complaint.

LEARN HOW TO
TURN ERRORS INTO AMENDS

In moral theory, restitution of an injury caused by a past transgression can be achieved by recognizing the injury, acknowledging one's wrongdoing, and making amends by taking steps to correct the past action, monitor present actions, and modify future actions. In ethical practice, the overarching ethical principle of *nonmaleficence* is concerned with avoiding harm to others. APA (2002) Ethical Standard 3.04 (Avoiding Harm) states, "Psychologists take reasonable steps to avoid harming their clients/patients, students, supervisees, research participants, organizational clients, and others with whom they work, and to minimize harm when it is foreseeable and unavoidable" (p. 1065).

Mistakes happen. Because correcting a mistake may sometimes ameliorate a situation in which a complaint has been filed, be sure to explain any actions that were taken to avoid or minimize harm to the client or others. From a risk-management perspective, there are occasions in which correcting a mistake can sometimes turn a potentially negative situation into a positive one. In their discussion of diversity issues in training group workers, G. Corey et al. (2007) state, "The ability to recover from mistakes gracefully is more important than not making any mistakes" (p. 468).

SHOW CONCERN FOR
YOUR CLIENT'S WELFARE

Just as a good client record shows that you are a careful and conscientious clinician, a good peer review response demonstrates that your behavior exemplifies "the three Cs." In other words, show you are a caring, concerned, and conscientious practitioner. When reviewing your written response to an ethics complaint investigation, your peers on the licensing board may read between the lines for indications that your actions and decisions demonstrated appropriate concern for the welfare of your client and others. Gutheil (1980) recommends that one's notes reflect active concern for the client's welfare.

NOTE ANY PEER CONSULTATIONS

Sooner or later, everyone faces a situation in which one's best efforts can result in adverse consequences. In such situations, one of the best defenses for one's actions is to have already obtained and documented consultation with a colleague (Doverspike, 1997c, 1999c). Peer consultation means talking with a respected colleague who is impartial, objective, and knowledgeable. Documentation of such consultation will at least demonstrate careful consideration of appropriate standards of care. Reasonableness of behavior is of utmost importance in making ethical decisions (Behnke, 2004). Ethically responsible behavior is based on the assumption of a reasonable *effort*. A practitioner who has documented that he or she has obtained a peer consultation on a case is a practitioner who has provided some evidence that he or she was striving for a reasonable standard of care. If your actions or decisions in a case were guided in part by consultation with a colleague, be sure to mention such consultation in your response. In fact, collegial consultations and good documentation are the two primary practices "that will most dramatically reduce the chances of successful malpractice suits" (R. L. Bednar et al., 1991, p. 59).

THINK IN TERMS OF
ASPIRATIONAL BEHAVIOR

Aspirational obligations represent ideals or the ethical "ceiling" of behavior whereas mandatory requirements represent minimal standards or the "floor" of ethical behavior (Haas & Malouf, 2005, p. 4). Aspirational ethical obligations represent the ideal achievement of excellence embodied in the general Ethical Principles contained in the APA *Ethical Principles of Psychologists and Code of Conduct* (2002). In contrast, mandatory requirements represent the enforceable Ethical Standards delineated in the more specific Code of Conduct section of the APA *Ethical Principles of Psychologists and Code of Conduct* (2002). When responding to an ethics investigation, think how your actions and decisions should reflect an aspirational level of behavior.

BE AWARE OF
PROCEDURES AND DEADLINES

Remember that it is important to comply with procedural deadlines. In most cases, one's first notification of a complaint may come in the form of a certified letter explaining the complaint and requesting a written response within a specified time period. A careful and conscientious practitioner responds within the time period, or requests an extension of time before the deadline has passed. A practitioner who responds a day or two after the deadline may give the impression that he or she is not concerned with such details, which may raise concern that he or she may not be a conscientious practitioner. If you cannot meet a deadline requirement, it is better to ask for an extension *before* rather than *after* the deadline has passed.

UNDERSTAND THE COMMITTEE FINDINGS

Known in some states as a "Finding of No Violation," some version of the following form letter is often the practitioner's last formal notice that an ethics investigation has been closed. With the exception of dismissing a complaint before an investigation even begins, this letter often represents one of the most favorable outcomes of a complaint that has been successfully resolved and closed:

Dear Reader:

The Board has concluded its investigation of the complaint filed against you. After careful consideration of the results of the investigation, the Board voted to close the case based on its determination that there was insufficient evidence that a violation of the laws and rules of the Board had occurred.

By closing this case, the Board is not making a clinical judgment as to the validity of the complaint. Rather, the Board made a determination, based on a thorough evaluation of the material presented to the Board, that there was insufficient proof of a significant violation of the laws and/or rules that would support further action by the Board.

We thank you for your cooperation in this manner. If you have any questions, please contact the Board office.

Sincerely yours,

Board Member

TURN A NEGATIVE
INTO A POSITIVE

The final stage of the resolution of an ethics complaint resolution should involve making some sense of it all. Regardless of the results of an investigation, cynicism does not have to be a final outcome. After the resolution and closure of the investigation, the next step is to take the "unpleasant experience" and learn from it, gain insight into yourself, and grow in your understanding of others. To use an old adage, "Experience is what we get when we don't get what we want."

One's ultimate goal in this regard would be to make some *meaning* of what has happened, and transform the circumstances into something positive. In the words of Aldous Huxley (1932), "Experience is not what happens to you, it is what you *do* with what happens to you." In my own way of thinking, "experience is not only what happens to us; it is what happens *within* us (Doverspike, 2005a, p. 279). Turning a minus into a plus is not simply a mathematical operation or a cognitive-behavioral technique, but rather it is a spiritual process in which someone takes a terrible experience and transforms it into something positive and meaningful.

SUMMARY OF RESPONDING
TO ETHICS COMPLAINTS

Mistakes happen. Good motives can lead to bad results. A clinician may be faced with a situation in which one's actions must be explained in response to a formal complaint. Given the amount of resources that are required to resolve complaints, it is important to take all client dissatisfactions seriously. When client dissatisfactions do arise to the level of a formal complaint, it is important to explain what happened in terms of specific details, behaviors, and events. An ideal response should show a careful decision-making process or a coherent rationale for one's actions. Regardless of the outcome of an ethics complaint, the unpleasant experience of an investigation can be beneficial if one can gain insight, grow in understanding others, and transform the circumstances into something positive. Keep in mind that good judgment comes from experience, and experience often comes from bad judgment. Remember that experience is not only what happens to you; it is what happens *within* you.

POINTS TO REMEMBER

- Remember there is no such thing as a frivolous complaint.
- Be a colleague, not an adversary.
- Be a good behaviorist when explaining details.
- Be able to explain what you did and why you did it.
- Learn not to blame the client.
- Learn how to turn errors into amends.
- Show concern for your client's welfare.
- Be able to note any peer consultations.
- Think in terms of aspirational behavior.
- Be aware of procedures and deadlines.
- Understand the committee findings.
- Turn negative events into positive experiences.

References

Ackerman, M. J., & Ackerman, M. C. (1997). Custody evaluation practices: A study of experienced professionals (revisited). *Professional Psychology: Research and Practice, 28*(2), 137-145.

Acuff, C., Bennett, B. E., Bricklin, P. M., Canter, M. B., Knapp, S. J., Moldawski, S., & Phelps, R. (1999). Considerations for ethical practice of managed care. *Professional Psychology: Research and Practice, 30*(6), 563-575.

American Association for Marriage and Family Therapy. (2001). *AAMFT Code of Ethics*. Washington, DC: Author.

American Counseling Association. (1999). *Ethical Standards for Internet On-Line Counseling*. Alexandria, VA: Author.

American Counseling Association. (2005). *Code of Ethics*. Alexandria, VA: Author.

American Home Assurance Company. (1990). *Psychologist's Professional Liability Policy*. New York: Author.

American Medical Association. (2006). *Physicians' Current Procedural Terminology*. Chicago: Author.

American Psychiatric Association. (2000). *Diagnostic and Statistical Manual of Mental Disorders* (4th ed. text rev.). Washington, DC: Author.

American Psychiatric Association. (2001). *The Principles of Medical Ethics With Annotations Especially Applicable to Psychiatry*. Washington, DC: Author.

American Psychological Association. (1981). Ethical principles of psychologists. *American Psychologist, 36*, 633-638.

American Psychological Association. (1987). *General Guidelines for Providers of Psychological Services*. Washington, DC: Author.

American Psychological Association. (1990). Ethical principles of psychologists (Amended June 2, 1989). *American Psychologist, 45*, 390-395.

American Psychological Association. (1992). Ethical principles of psychologists and code of conduct. *American Psychologist, 47*, 1597-1611.

American Psychological Association. (1993). Record keeping guidelines. *American Psychologist, 48*, 984-986.

American Psychological Association. (1994). Guidelines for child custody evaluations in divorce proceedings. *American Psychologist, 49*(7), 677-680.

American Psychological Association. (1996). Rules and procedures. Ethics Committee of the American Psychological Association. *American Psychologist, 51*(5), 529-548.

American Psychological Association. (2002). Ethical principles of psychologists and code of conduct. *American Psychologist, 57*(12), 1060-1073.

American Psychological Association. (2007). *Record Keeping Guidelines.* Retrieved March 22, 2007, from http://www.apa.org/practice/recordkeeping.pdf

American Psychological Association Committee on Professional Practice and Standards. (1999). Guidelines for psychological evaluations in child protection matters. *American Psychologist, 54*, 586-593.

American Psychological Association Division 12 Section II (Section on Clinical Geropsychology) and Division 20 (Adult Development and Aging) Interdivisional Task Force on Practice of Clinical Geropsychology. (2003). *Guidelines for Psychological Practice With Older Adults.* Washington, DC: Author.

American Psychological Association Division 44/Committee on Lesbian, Gay, and Bisexual Concerns Task Force on Guidelines for Psychotherapy With Lesbian, Gay, and Bisexual Clients. (2000). Psychotherapy with lesbian, gay, and bisexual clients. *American Psychologist, 55*, 1440-1451.

American Psychological Association Insurance Trust, Professional Liability Insurance Program. (1996). *Professional Liability Insurance for Psychologists. Application Form.* Des Moines, IA: Author.

American Psychological Association Office of Ethnic Minority Affairs. (1993). Guidelines for providers of psychological services to ethnic, linguistic, and culturally diverse populations. *American Psychologist, 48*, 45-48.

American Psychological Association Practice Organization. (2002). *Getting Ready for HIPAA: A Primer for Psychologists.* Washington, DC: Author.

American Psychological Association Practice Organization. (2003). *HIPAA for Psychologists.* Washington, DC: Author.

American Psychological Association Presidential Task Force on the Assessment of Age-Consistent Memory Decline and Dementia. (1998). Guidelines for the evaluation of dementia and age-related cognitive decline. *American Psychologist, 53*, 1298-1303.

American Psychological Association Task Force on Sex Bias and Sex Role Stereotyping in Psychotherapeutic Practice. (1978). Guidelines for therapy with women. *American Psychologist, 33*, 1122-1123.

Anders, P. B., & Terrell, C. J. (2006). Tarasoff trends impact therapists. *Georgia Psychologist, 60*(2), 15.

Anderson, B. S. (1996). *The Counselor and the Law* (4th ed.). Alexandria, VA: American Counseling Association.

Anderson, M. (2005). *Informed Consent for Special Circumstances.* Form distributed at a meeting of the Ethics Committee, Georgia Psychological Association, Atlanta, GA.

Andrews, L. B. (1984). Informed consent statutes and the decision-making process. *Journal of Legal Medicine, 5,* 163-217.

Baird, K. A. (2001). How to respond to patient special requests to step outside of traditional therapeutic boundaries: Psychologists who practice in metropolitan areas. *Georgia Psychologist, 55*(2), 23-24.

Barnett, J. E. (1997). How to avoid malpractice. *The Independent Practitioner, 17*(1), 20-22.

Barth, J. T. (2000). Commentary on "Disclosure of Tests and Raw Test Data to the Courts" by Paul Lees-Haley and John Courtney. *Neuropsychology Review, 10*(3), 179-180.

Beauchamp, T. L., & Childress, J. F. (2001). *Principles of Biomedical Ethics* (5th ed.). New York: Oxford University Press.

Bednar, R. L., Bednar, S. C., Lambert, M. J., & Waite, D. R. (1991). *Psychotherapy With High-Risk Clients: Legal and Professional Standards.* Pacific Grove, CA: Brooks/ Cole.

Behnke, S. (2004). Multiple relationships and APA's new ethics code: Values and applications. *Monitor on Psychology, 35*(1), 66-68.

Behnke, S. (2005, October 8). *Ethical Decision-Making for Mental Health Professionals.* Ethics workshop presented to the Georgia Psychological Association, Atlanta, GA.

Behnke, S., Preis, J. J., & Bates, R. T. (1998). *The Essentials of California Mental Health Law.* New York: Norton.

Bennett, B. E., Bricklin, P. M., Harris, E., Knapp, S., VandeCreek, L., & Younggren, J. N. (2006). *Assessing and Managing Risk in Psychological Practice: An Individualized Approach.* Rockville, MD: The Trust.

Bennett, B. E., Bryant, B. K., VandenBos, G. R., & Greenwood, A. (1990). *Professional Liability and Risk Management.* Washington, DC: American Psychological Association.

Bennett, B., Harris, E., & Remar, R. (1995, April 22-23). *Risk Management.* APAIT ethics workshop presented at the annual meeting of the Georgia Psychological Association, Atlanta, GA.

Bennett, B., Harris, E., & Remar, R. (1996, May 30). *Ethics and Risk Management.* APAIT ethics workshop presented at the annual meeting of the Georgia Psychological Association, Savannah, GA.

Bennett, B., Harris, E., & Remar, R. (1997, May 15). *Ethics and Risk Management.* APAIT ethics workshop presented at the annual meeting of the Georgia Psychological Association, Atlanta, GA.

Bentham, J. (1948). *An Introduction to the Principles of Morals and Legislation*. New York: Hafar Publishing. (Original work published 1863)

Berkowitz, L. (1968). Impulse, aggression, and the gun. *Psychology Today, 2*(September), 19-22.

Berkowitz, L. (1974). Some determinants of impulsive aggression: Role of mediated associations with reinforcements for aggression. *Psychological Review, 81*, 165-176.

Berkowitz, L., & LePage, A. (1967). Weapons as aggression eliciting stimuli. *Journal of Personality and Social Psychology, 7*, 202-207.

Bersoff, D. N. (2003). *Ethical Conflicts in Psychology* (3rd ed.). Washington, DC: American Psychological Association.

Borys, D. S., & Pope, K. S. (1989). Dual Relationships Between Therapist and Client: A National Study of Psychologists, Psychiatrists, and Social Workers. *Professional Psychology: Research and Practice, 20*(5), 283-293.

Bradley Center, Inc. v. Wessner, et al., 161 Ga. App. 576 (287 SE 2d 716) (1982).

Bridge, P. J., & Bascue, L. O. (1988). A record form for psychotherapy supervisors. In P. A. Keller & S. R. Heyman (Eds.), *Innovations in Clinical Practice: A Source Book* (Vol. 7, pp. 331-336). Sarasota, FL: Professional Resource Exchange.

Buchanan, W. (1997, January 17). *Mental Health Ethics and Georgia Law*. Continuing education workshop sponsored by the Georgia School of Professional Psychology at Georgia State University, North Campus, Atlanta, GA.

Buckley, P., Karasu, T. B., & Charles, E. (1981). Psychotherapists view their personal therapy. *Psychotherapy: Theory, Research, and Practice, 18*(3), 299-305.

California Civil Code, Section 43.92 (1985).

Campbell, E., & Webb, C. (2004). Commentary from the Licensing Board. *Georgia Psychologist, Vol. 58*(1), 7.

Campbell, L., Doverspike, W. F., Meck, D., McIntyre, T., & Sauls, M. (1999, May 15). *Lessons Learned: Educating Psychologists and Protecting the Public*. Ethics workshop presented at the annual meeting of the Georgia Psychological Association, Emory Conference Center, Atlanta, GA.

Canadian Psychological Association. (2000). *Canadian Code of Ethics for Psychologists* (3rd ed.). Ottawa, Ontario, Canada: Author.

Canter, M. B., Bennett, B. E., Jones, S. E., & Nagy, T. F. (1994). *Ethics for Psychologists: A Commentary on the APA Ethics Code*. Washington, DC: American Psychological Association.

Canterbury v. Spence, 464 F.2d 772, 789 (D.C. Cir. 1972).

Clites v. Iowa, No. 46247 (Pottawattamie County, Iowa, 1980).

Cobia, D. C., & Boes, S. R. (2000). Professional disclosure statements and formal plans for supervision: Two strategies for minimizing the risk of ethical conflicts in postmaster's supervision. *Journal of Counseling and Development, 78*(3), 293-296.

Committee on Ethical Guidelines for Forensic Psychologists. (1991). Specialty Guidelines for Forensic Psychologists. *Law and Human Behavior, 15*(6), 655-665.

Corey, G., Corey, M., & Callanan, M. (2003). *Issues and Ethics in the Helping Professions* (6th ed.). Pacific Grove, CA: Brooks/Cole.

Corey, G., Corey, M., & Callanan, M. (2007). *Issues and Ethics in the Helping Professions* (7th ed.). Pacific Grove, CA: Brooks/ Cole.

Crawford, R. J. (1994). *Avoiding Counselor Malpractice*. Alexandria, VA: American Counseling Association.

DeFilippis, N. A., Wilbanks, M., Doverspike, W. F., Dsurney, J., & Bridges, J. D. (1997, February 14). *Everyday Considerations in Treating Litigating Clients: An Ethical Balancing Act.* Workshop presented at the Georgia Psychological Association Central Office, Atlanta, GA.

Dilts, R. (1983). *Applications of Neuro-Linguistic Programming*. Cupertino, CA: Meta Publications.

Donaldson v. O'Connor, 493 F. 2d 507 (5th Cir. 1974).

Doverspike, W. F. (1995). Some survival tips for dealing with insurance companies and managed care. In L. VandeCreek, S. Knapp, & T. L. Jackson (Eds.), *Innovations in Clinical Practice: A Source Book* (Vol. 14, pp. 255-262). Sarasota, FL: Professional Resource Press.

Doverspike, W. F. (1996a). Informed consent for psychological services: Clinical services. *Georgia Psychologist, 50*(2), 56-58.

Doverspike, W. F. (1996b). Informed consent for psychological services: Financial responsibility. *Georgia Psychologist, 50*(4), 24-26.

Doverspike, W. F. (1997a). Ethical decision making: Doing the next right thing. *Georgia Psychologist, 51*(2), 29-33.

Doverspike, W. F. (1997b). Informed consent forms. In L. VandeCreek, S. Knapp, & T. L. Jackson (Eds.), *Innovations in Clinical Practice: A Source Book* (Vol. 15, pp. 201-214). Sarasota, FL: Professional Resource Press.

Doverspike, W. F. (1997c). Putting ethics into practice: Some personal reflections. *Georgia Psychologist, 51*(1), 22-24.

Doverspike, W. F. (1999a). Consulting with colleagues. *Georgia Psychologist, 53*(4), 27-28.

Doverspike, W. F. (1999b). *Ethical Risk Management: Guidelines for Practice*. Sarasota, FL: Professional Resource Press.

Doverspike, W. F. (1999c). Ethical risk management: Protecting your practice. In L. VandeCreek & T. L. Jackson (Eds.), *Innovations in Clinical Practice: A Source Book* (Vol. 17, pp. 269-278). Sarasota, FL: Professional Resource Press.

Doverspike, W. F. (1999d). *Multiaxial Diagnostic Inventory - Revised (MDI-R)*. Sarasota, FL: Professional Resource Press.

Doverspike, W. F. (1999e). You've got mail: How to respond to an ethics complaint. *Georgia Psychologist, 53*(2), 25-27.

Doverspike, W. F. (2000). Aspiring to excellence. *Georgia Psychologist, 54*(2), 6.

Doverspike, W. (2001). Common ethical concerns of psychologists. *Georgia Psychologist, 55*(4), 15-19.

Doverspike, W. (2003a). The 2002 APA Ethics Code: An overview. *Georgia Psychologist, 57*(1), 27-32.

Doverspike, W. (2003b). [Review of the book *A Guide to the 2002 Revision of the American Psychological Association's Ethics Code*]. *Georgia Psychologist, 57*(2), 25-26.

Doverspike, W. (2004a). Boundary violations and psychotherapy [Review of the book *Dual Relationships and Psychotherapy*]. *Contemporary Psychology, 49*(2), 209-211.

Doverspike, W. (2004b). A brief history of child protection legislation: From 1874 to 2004. *Georgia Psychologist, 58*(1), 2-3.

Doverspike, W. F. (2004c, December 17). *Case Consultations With Colleagues.* Ethics workshop presented to Georgia Psychological Association, GPA Central Office, Atlanta, GA.

Doverspike, W. F. (2005a). Confessions of a secular priest: A story of faith turned inside out. *Journal of Psychology and Christianity, 24*(3), 278-280.

Doverspike, W. F. (2005b, December 2). *Consulting With Colleagues: Interactive Discussion of Common Ethical Dilemmas.* Ethics workshop presented at the Central Office of the Georgia Psychological Association, Atlanta, GA.

Doverspike, W. (2005c). Ethical considerations in keeping psychological records of children. *Georgia Psychologist, 59*(2), 25.

Doverspike, W. (2005d). The ethics of record-keeping: Psychotherapy notes and progress notes. *Georgia Psychologist, 59*(3), 21.

Doverspike, W. F. (2006a, December 8). *Consulting With Colleagues: Fall Seminar.* Ethics workshop presented at the Central Office of the Georgia Psychological Association, Atlanta, GA.

Doverspike, W. (2006b). The ethics of record-keeping: Discharge summaries and disclosures. *Georgia Psychologist, 60*(1), 13-14.

Doverspike, W. (2006c). The ethics of record-keeping: Risk managed notes and record summaries. *Georgia Psychologist, 60*(1), 13-14.

Doverspike, W. (2006d). Psychology and the law. *Georgia Psychologist, 60*(2), 2.

Doverspike, W. F. (2007). The so-called duty to warn: Protecting the public versus protecting the patient. *Georgia Psychologist, 61*(3), 20.

Doverspike, W. F., & Stone, A. V. (2000, June 16). *Duty to Protect: How Far Are You Prepared to Go?* Ethics workshop presented to the Georgia Psychological Association, Atlanta, GA.

Eberlein, L. (1987). Introducing ethics to beginning psychologists: A problem-solving approach. *Professional Psychology: Research and Practice, 18,* 353-359.

Ebert, B. W. (2006). *Multiple Relationships and Conflict of Interest forMental Health Professionals: A Conservative Psycholegal Approach.* Sarasota, FL: Professional Resource Press.

Ellis, E. (2006). Ten ethical pitfalls to avoid when doing child and family forensic work. *Georgia Psychologist, 60*(2), 12-14.

Ewing v. Goldstein, 120 Cal.App.4th 807 (2d App. Dist. 2004).

Eyde, L. D., & Quaintance, M. K. (1988). Ethical issues and cases in the practice of personnel psychology. *Professional Psychology: Research and Practice, 19,* 148-154.

Fleer, J. I. (1999). The myth of risk management. *Independent Practitioner, 19,* 57.

Florida Statutes. State of Florida Chapter 21U-15.004. New 6-23-82. Amended 12-21-86.

Florida Statutes (490.0111). (Formerly 21U-15.004, amended 05-14-01). *Sexual Misconduct in the Practice of Psychology.* Chapter 64B19-16.003 (Florida Administrative Code, Psychology) Specific Authority.

Florida Statutes. State of Florida Chapter 39.201 (1[a]). "Reporting Child Abuse." (2005).

Florida Statutes. State of Florida Chapter 415.101. "Adult Protected Services Act." (2003).

Freudenberger, H. J. (1980). *Burnout: How to Beat the High Cost of Success.* New York: Bantam Books.

Gabbard, G. O. (1994). Teetering on the precipice: A commentary on Lazarus's "How certain boundaries and ethics diminish therapeutic effectiveness." *Ethics and Behavior, 4*(3), 283-286.

Gabbard, G. O., & Pope, K. (1988). Sexual intimacies after termination: Clinical, ethical, and legal aspects. *The Independent Practitioner, 8*(2), 21-26.

Garcia, J., Cartwright, B., Winston, S. M., & Borzuchowska, B. (2003). Transcultural integrative model for ethical decision-making. *Journal of Counseling and Development, 81,* 268-277.

Garner v. Stone, No. 97A-320250-1 (Ga., DeKalb County Super. Ct. Dec. 16, 1999).

Georgia Psychological Association. (1996). *Rules and Procedures of The Georgia Psychological Association Ethics Committee (Revised June 18, 1996).* Atlanta, GA: Author.

Gibson, W. T., & Pope, K. S. (1993). The ethics of counseling: A national survey of certified counselors. *Journal of Counseling and Development, 71*(3), 330-336.

Golden, L. (2002). Authorization to continue: A posttermination friendship evolves. In A. A. Lazarus & O. Zur (Eds.), *Dual Relationships and Psychotherapy* (pp. 409-422). New York: Springer.

Good Communication Is a Key Factor in Avoiding Malpractice Suits. Press Release, February 18, 1997. Agency for Healthcare Research and Quality, Rockville, MD. Retrieved June 1, 2007, from http://www.ahrq.gov/news/press/malpract.htm

Gottlieb, M. C. (1993). Avoiding exploitive dual relationships: A decision-making model. *Psychotherapy, 30,* 41-48.

Greenberg, S. A., & Shuman, D. W. (1997). Irreconcilable conflict between therapeutic and forensic roles. *Professional Psychology: Research and Practice, 28*(1), 50-57.

Greenson, R. R. (1967). *The Technique and Practice of Psychoanalysis.* New York: International Universities Press.

Gutheil, T. G. (1980). Paranoia and progress notes: A guide to forensically informed psychiatric record keeping. *Hospital and Community Psychiatry, 13,* 479-482.

Gutheil, T. G., & Gabbard, G. O. (1993). The concept of boundaries in clinical practice: Theoretical and risk management dimensions. *American Journal of Psychiatry, 150*(2), 188-196.

Haas, L. J., & Malouf, J. L. (2005). *Keeping Up the Good Work: A Practitioner's Guide to Mental Health Ethics* (4th ed.). Sarasota, FL: Professional Resource Press.

Hall, J. S. (1998). *Deepening the Treatment.* Northvale, NJ: Jason Aronson.

Handelsman, M. M., & Galvin, M. D. (1988). Facilitating informed consent for outpatient psychotherapy: A suggested written format. *Professional Psychology: Research and Practice, 19,* 223-225.

Harrar, W. R., VandeCreek, L., & Knapp, S. (1990). Ethical and legal aspects of clinical supervision. *Professional Psychology: Research and Practice, 21*(1), 37-41.

Harris, E. (2004, May 13). *APAIT Workshop: Part I: Legal and Ethical Risk Management in Professional Psychological Practice.* APAIT ethics workshop presented at the annual meeting of the Georgia Psychological Association, Hilton Head Island, SC.

Harris, E., & Remar, R. (1998, June 5). *Ethics and Risk Management.* APAIT ethics workshop presented to the Georgia Psychological Association, Atlanta, GA.

Health Insurance Portability and Accountability Act. Public Law 104-191. (1996). Available at www.access.gpo.gov/nara/cfr/index.html

Herlihy, B., & Corey, G. (1996). *American Counseling Association Ethical Standards Casebook* (5th ed.). Alexandria, VA: American Counseling Association.

Herlihy, B., & Corey, G. (1997). *Boundary Issues in Counseling: Multiple Roles and Responsibilities.* Alexandria, VA: American Counseling Association.

Herlihy, B., & Corey, G. (2006). *American Counseling Association Ethical Standards Casebook* (6th ed.). Alexandria, VA: American Counseling Association.

Herman, J. L., Gartrell, N., Olarte, S., Feldstein, M., & Localio, R. (1987). Psychiatrist-patient sexual contact: Results of a national survey, II: Psychiatrists' attitudes. *American Journal of Psychiatry, 144*, 164-169.

Hickson, G. B., Federspiel, C. F., Pichert, J. W., Miller, C. S., Gauld-Jaeger, J., & Bost, P. (2002). Patient complaints and malpractice risk. *Journal of the American Medical Association, 287*(22), 2951-2957.

Hill, M. (1999). Barter: Ethical considerations in psychotherapy. *Women and Therapy, 22*(3), 81-91.

Hill, M., Glaser, K., & Harden, J. (1995). A feminist model for ethical decision making. In E. J. Rave & C. C. Larsen (Eds.), *Ethical Decision Making in Therapy: Feminist Perspectives* (pp. 18-37). New York: Guilford.

Homan, M. (2004). *Promoting Community Change: Making It Happen in the Real World* (3rd ed.). Belmont, CA: Brooks/Cole-Wadsworth.

Huxley, A. L. (1932). *Texts and Pretexts: An Anthology With Commentaries.* London: Chatto & Windus.

Hyman, S. M. (2002). The shirtless jock therapist and the bikini-clad client: An exploration of chance extratherapeutic encounters. In A. A. Lazarus & O. Zur (Eds.), *Dual Relationships and Psychotherapy* (pp. 348-359). New York: Springer.

In the Matter of the Accusation Against Leon Jerome Oziel, Ph.D. (1986). Board of Psychology, State of California. Case No. D-3205.

Jablonski v. United States, 712 F.2d 391 (9th Cir. 1983).

Jaffee v. Redmond, WL 315 841 (US 1996).

Jourard, S. M. (1971). *The Transparent Self.* New York: D. Van Nostrand.

Kachigian, C., & Felthous, A. R. (2004). Court responses to Tarasoff statutes. *Journal of the American Academy of Psychiatry and the Law, 32*(3), 263-274.

Kalichman, S. C. (1993). Mandated reporting of suspected child abuse. *Ethics, Law, and Policy.* Washington, DC: American Psychological Association.

Kalichman, S. C., & Craig, M. E. (1991). Professional psychologists' decisions to report suspected child abuse: Clinician and situation influences. *Professional Psychology: Research and Practice, 22*(1), 84-89.

Kant, I. (2002). *Groundwork for the Metaphysics of Morals* (A. W. Wood, Trans.). New Haven, CT: Yale University Press. (Original work published 1785)

Keeping Children and Families Safe Act of 2003, Pub. L. 108-36, 42 U.S.C. § 5101 *et seq.* (2003).

Keith-Spiegel, P., & Koocher, G. P. (1985). *Ethics in Psychology: Professional Standards and Cases.* New York: Random House.

Kilburn, R. B., Nathan, P. E., & Thoreson, R. W. (Eds). (1986). *Professionals in Distress: Issues, Syndromes, and Solutions in Psychology.* Washington, DC: American Psychological Association.

Kingsbury, S. J. (1987). Cognitive differences between clinical psychologists and psychiatrists. *American Psychologist, 42,* 152-156.

Kirkland, K., Kirkland, K. L., & Reaves, R. P. (2004). On the professional use of disciplinary data. *Professional Psychology: Research and Practice, 35*(2), 179-184.

Kitchener, K. S. (1984). Intuition, critical evaluation and ethical principles: The foundation for ethical decisions in counseling psychology. *The Counseling Psychologist, 12,* 306-310.

Knapp, S., & VandeCreek, L. (1997). Questions and answers about clinical supervision. In L. VandeCreek, S. Knapp, & T. L. Jackson (Eds.), *Innovations in Clinical Practice: A Source Book* (Vol. 15, pp. 189-197). Sarasota, FL: Professional Resource Press.

Koocher, G. P., & Keith-Spiegel, P. (1998). *Ethics in Psychology: Professional Standards and Cases* (2nd ed.). New York: Oxford Textbooks in Clinical Psychology.

Kovacs, A. L. (1984). The increasing malpractice exposure of psychologists. *The Independent Practitioner, 4*(2), 12-14.

Ladany, N., Lehrman-Waterman, D., Molinaro, M., & Wolgast, B. (1999). Psychotherapy supervisor ethical practices: Adherence to guidelines, the supervisory working alliance, and supervisee satisfaction. *The Counseling Psychologist, 27*(3) 443-475.

Lankton, S. (1980). *Practical Magic: A Translation of Basic Neuro-Linguistic Programming into Clinical Psychotherapy.* Cuperton, CA: Meta Publications.

Lawrence, G., & Robinson-Kurpius, S. E. (2000). Legal and ethical issues involved when counseling minors in nonschool settings. *Journal of Counseling and Development, 78*(2), 130-137.

Lazarus, A. A. (2001). Not all "dual relationships" are taboo: Some need to enhance treatment outcomes. *The National Psychologist, (10)*1, 16.

Lazarus, A. A. (2002). How certain boundaries and ethics diminish therapeutic effectiveness. In A. A. Lazarus & O. Zur (Eds.), *Dual Relationships and Psychotherapy* (pp. 25-31). New York: Springer.

Lazarus, A. A., & Zur, O. (Eds.). (2002). *Dual Relationships and Psychotherapy.* New York: Springer.

Lees-Haley, P. R., & Courtney, J. C. (2000a). Disclosure of tests and raw test data to the courts: A need for reform. *Neuropsychology Review, 10*(3), 169-174.

Lees-Haley, P. R., & Courtney, J. C. (2000b). Reply to the commentary on "Disclosure of tests and raw test data to the courts." *Neuropsychology Review, 10*(3), 181-182.

Levinson, W., Gorawara-Bhat, R., & Lamb, J. (2000). A study of patient clues and physician responses in primary care and surgical settings. *Journal of the American Medical Association, 284*(8), 1021-1027.

Levinson, W., Roter, D. L., Mullooly, J. P., Dull, V. T., & Frankel, R. M. (1997). Physician-patient communication. The relationship with malpractice claims among primary care physicians and surgeons. *Journal of the American Medical Association, 277*(7), 553-559.

Linehan, M. M. (1987a). *Cognitive Behavioral Treatment of Borderline Personality Disorder.* New York: Guilford.

Linehan, M. M. (1987b). Dialectical behavior therapy for borderline personality disorder: Theory and method. *Bulletin of the Menninger Clinic, 51,* 261-276.

Livermore, J., Malmquist, C., & Meehl, P. (1968). On the justification for civil commitment. *University of Pennsylvania Law Review, 117,* 75-96.

Magellan Behavioral Health. (1999). *Documentation Standards for Behavior Treatment Records.* Maryland Heights, MO: Author.

Maheu, M. M. (2001). Practicing psychotherapy on the internet: Risk management challenges and opportunities. *The Register Report, 27,* 23-28.

Marlatt, G. A. (1985). Relapse prevention: A general overview. In G. A. Marlatt & J. R. Gordon (Eds.), *Relapse Prevention: Maintenance Strategies in the Treatment of Addictive Behaviors* (pp. 3-16). New York: Guilford.

McCullough, J. P., Jr. (2000). *Treatment for Chronic Depression: Cognitive Behavioral Analysis System of Psychotherapy (CBASP).* New York: Guilford.

McGarrah, N. A. (2001). Reporting child abuse: The psychologist's dilemma. *Georgia Psychologist, 55*(1), 28-29.

McMinn, M. R., & Meek, K. R. (1996). Ethics among Christian counselors: A survey of beliefs and behaviors. *Journal of Psychology and Theology, 24,* 26-37.

McMinn, M. R., Meek, K. R., & McRay, B. W. (1997). Beliefs and behaviors among CAPS members regarding ethical issues. *Journal of Psychology and Christianity, 16*(1), 18-35.

Meara, N. M., Schmidt, L. D., & Day, J. D. (1996). Principles and virtues: A foundation for ethical decisions, policies, and character. *The Counseling Psychologist, 24*(1), 4-77.

Mill, J. S. (2001). *Utilitarianism* (2nd ed.; G. Sher, Ed.). Indianapolis: Hackett Publishing Company. (Original work published 1863)

Monahan, J. (1981). *Predicting Violent Behavior: An Assessment of Clinical Techniques.* Beverly Hills, CA: Sage.

Monahan, J. (1993). Limiting therapist exposure to Tarasoff liability. *American Psychologist, 48*(3), 242-250.

Moore, G. (1900). *The Bending of the Bough: A Comedy in Five Acts, Act IV.* New York: H. S. Stone.

Morris, R. J. (1997). Child custody evaluations: A risky business. *Register Report, 23*(1), 6-7.

Myers, J. E., Sweeney, T. J., & Witmer, J. M. (2000). The wheel of wellness counseling for wellness: A holistic model. *Journal of Counseling and Development, 78*(3), 251-266.

National Association of Social Workers. (1999). *Code of Ethics.* Washington, DC: Author.

National Child Abuse Prevention and Treatment Act of 1974, Pub. L. No. 93-247, 42 U.S.C. § 5101 *et seq.* (1974).

North Carolina Society for Clinical Social Work. (2000). *A Suggested Model for the Sudden Termination of a Clinical Social Work Practice.* Durham, NC: Author.

Official Code of Georgia Annotated § 19-7-5 (1999 & amended 2006), "Reporting of Child Abuse."

Official Code of Georgia Annotated § 31-33-2 (1981), "Furnishing Copy of Records to Patient, Provider, or Other Authorized Person."

Official Code of Georgia Annotated § 31-33-2 (1981 & amended 2006), "Furnishing Copy of Records to Patient, Provider, or Other Authorized Person."

Official Code of Georgia Annotated § 31-33-4 (1981 & amended 1985), "Mental Health Records."

Official Code of Georgia Annotated § 49-5-40 (1975 & amended 1993), "Definitions; Confidentiality of Records; Restricted Access to Records."

Othmer, E. O., & Othmer, S. C. (1989). *The Clinical Interview Using DSM-III-R.* Washington, DC: American Psychiatric Press.

People v. Poddar, 10 Cal.3d 750, 758, 111 Cal.Rptr. 910, 518 P.2d 342 (1974).

Petrila, J. D., & Otto, R. K. (2003). *Law & Mental Health Professionals: Florida* (2nd ed.). Washington, DC: American Psychological Association.

Piazza, N. J., & Baruth, N. E. (1990). Client record guidelines. *Journal of Counseling and Development, 68*, 313-316.

Piazza, N. J., & Yeager, R. D. (1991). The client record as a tool for risk management. In P. A. Keller & S. R. Heyman (Eds.), *Innovations in Clinical Practice: A Source Book* (Vol. 10, pp. 341-352). Sarasota, FL: Professional Resource Exchange.

Pope, K. S. (1986). New trends in malpractice cases and changes in APA liability insurance. *The Independent Practitioner, 6*(4), 23-26.

Pope, K. S. (1989a). Malpractice suits, licensing disciplinary actions, and ethics cases: Frequencies, causes, and costs. *The Independent Practitioner, 9*(1), 22-26.

Pope, K. S. (1989b, February 4). *Reducing Risks of Ethical Violations and Malpractice.* Workshop presented at the Georgia Psychological Association Midwinter Conference, Hilton Head Island, SC.

Pope, K. S., Sonne, J. L., & Holroyd, J. (1993). *Sexual Feelings in Psychotherapy: Explorations for Therapists and Therapists-in-Training.* Washington, DC: American Psychological Association.

Pope, K. S., Tabachnick, B. G., & Keith-Spiegel, P. (1987). Ethics of practice: The beliefs and behaviors of psychologists as therapists. *American Psychologist, 42,* 993-1006.

Pope, K. S., & Vasquez, M. J. T. (1991). *Ethics in Psychotherapy and Counseling: A Practical Guide for Psychologists.* San Francisco: Jossey-Bass.

Pope, K. S., & Vasquez, M. J. T. (1998). *Ethics in Psychotherapy and Counseling: A Practical Guide for Psychologists* (2nd ed.). San Francisco: Jossey-Bass.

Pope, K. S., & Vasquez, M. J. T. (2005). *How to Survive and Thrive as a Therapist: Information, Ideas, and Resources for Psychologists in Practice.* Washington, DC: American Psychological Association.

Rabinowitz, E. E. (1991). The male-to-male embrace. Breaking the touch taboo in a men's therapy group. *Journal of Counseling and Development, 69*(6), 574-576.

Remar, R. (2000). *Proposed Code Section Establishing a Duty to Warn.* Unpublished manuscript.

Remar, R. B., & Hubert, R. N. (1996). *Law & Mental Health Professionals: Georgia.* Washington, DC: American Psychological Association.

Remley, T. P., & Herlihy, B. (2005). *Ethical, Legal, and Professional Issues in Counseling* (2nd ed.). Upper Saddle River, NJ: Merrill/ Prentice-Hall.

Rolf, I. P. (1989). *Rolfing: Reestablishing the Natural Alignment and Structural Integration of the Human Body for Vitality and Well-Being.* Rochester, VT: Healing Arts Press.

Rules of Georgia Composite Board of Professional Counselors, Social Workers, and Marriage and Family Therapists, Chapter 135-7-.03, "Confidentiality," Section 2[C], "Unprofessional conduct . . ." O.C.G.A. § 43-7A-5(d), adopted F. Feb. 28, 2000; eff. Mar. 19, 2000.

Rules of the State Board of Examiners of Psychologists, Chapter 510-2-.01, Section 2(c), "Application by Examination," adopted F. Mar. 18, 2004; eff. Apr. 7, 2004. O.C.G.A. § 43-39-12. 2004.

Rules of the State Board of Examiners of Psychologists, Chapter 510-3-.12(1a), "Violations of Applicable Statutes" (Original Rule entitled "Violations of Law," adopted F. Jul 27, 1994; eff. Aug. 16, 1994). O.G.G.A. § 43-1-19(a), 43-1-25, 43-39-5(d), 43-39-13. 1994.

Rules of the State Board of Examiners of Psychologists, Chapter 510-4-.02, "Code of Ethics," Section 4.05, "Disclosures," adopted F. Mar. 18, 2004; eff. Apr. 7, 2004. O.C.G.A. § 43-39-12. 2004.

Rules of the State Board of Examiners of Psychologists, Chapter 510-5, "Supplemental Code of Conduct," adopted F. Mar. 18, 2004; eff. Apr. 7, 2004. O.C.G.A. § 43-39-12. 2004.

Rules of the State Board of Examiners of Psychologists, Chapter 510-5-.02, "Definitions," adopted F. Mar. 18, 2004; eff. Apr. 7, 2004. O.C.G.A. § 43-39-12. 2004.

Rules of the State Board of Examiners of Psychologists, Chapter 510-5-.03, "Maintenance and Retention of Records," adopted F. July 27, 1994; eff. Aug. 16, 1994. O.C.G.A. § 43-39-12. 1994.

Rules of the State Board of Examiners of Psychologists, Chapter 510-5-.04, "Maintenance and Retention of Records," adopted F. Mar. 18, 2004; eff. Apr. 7, 2004. O.C.G.A. § 43-39-12. 2004.

Rules of the State Board of Examiners of Psychologists, Chapter 510-5-.05(1), "Dual Relationship Affecting Psychologist's Judgment," adopted F. July 27, 1994; eff. Aug. 16, 1994; rev. April 18, 1996. O.G.G.A. § 43-39-12. 1996.

Rules of the State Board of Examiner's of Psychologists, Chapter 510-5-.05(2), "Prohibited Dual Relationships," adopted F. Mar. 18, 2004; eff. Apr. 7, 2004. O.C.G.A. § 43-39-12. 2004.

Rules of the State Board of Examiners of Psychologists, Chapter 510-5-.06(3), "Delegation to and Supervision of Supervisees of Psychological Services," adopted F. Mar. 18, 2004; eff. Apr. 7, 2004. O.C.G.A. § 43-39-12. 2004.

St. Germaine, J. (1993). Dual relationships: What's wrong with them? *American Counselor, 2*(3), 25-30.

Sanders, R. K. (1997). *Christian Counseling Ethics: A Handbook for Therapists, Pastors, and Counselors.* Downers Grove, IL: InterVarsity Press.

Sauls, M., Kleemeier, C., Kleemeier, B., Phipps, A., & Doverspike, W. (2001). *GPA Psychologists' Toolbox: Strategies for Building and Maintaining a Successful Private Practice.* Atlanta, GA: Georgia Psychological Association.

Saxton, J. W., & Finkelstein, M. M. (2005). Reducing your risk of malpractice claims. *Physician's News Digest*, April 2005. Retrieved July 14, 2006, from http://www.physiciansnews.com/law/405saxton.html

Schaffer, S. J. (1997). Don't be aloof about record-keeping; it may be your best liability insurance. *The National Psychologist, 6*(1), 21.

Schlosser, B., & Tower, R. B. (1991). Office policies for assessment services. In P. A. Keller & S. R. Heyman (Eds.), *Innovations in Clinical Practice* (Vol. 10, pp. 393-411). Sarasota, FL: Professional Resource Exchange.

Schrader v. Kohut, 239 Ga. App. 134, 519 S.E. 2d 307 (1999).

Shapiro, D. (1994, January 15). *Ethical Constraints in an Age of Litigation.* Workshop presented at the Midwinter Conference, Georgia Psychological Association, Ashville, NC.

Shapiro, D. L. (2000). Commentary: Disclosure of tests and raw test data to the courts. *Neuropsychology Review, 10*(3), 175-176.

Sinclair, C., Poizner, S., Gilmour-Barrett, K., & Randall, D. (1987). The development of a code of ethics for Canadian psychologists. *Canadian Psychology, 28,* 1-8.

Smith, D., & Fitzpatrick, M. (1995). Patient-therapist boundary issues: An integrative review of theory and research. *Professional Psychology: Research and Practice, 26*(5), 499-506.

Smith, R., Graves, J., Hall, J., & Paddock, J. (1994, November 17). *Therapeutic Malpractice.* Continuing education workshop presented in Atlanta, GA.

Smith, R. S. (2003, January 24). *HIPAA: A Fast Overview.* Handout presented at the Georgia Psychological Association, Brasstown Valley Resort, GA.

Soisson, E. L., VandeCreek, L., & Knapp, S. (1987). Thorough record keeping: A good defense in a litigious era. *Professional Psychology: Research and Practice, 19*(5), 498-502.

Stadler, H. A. (1986). Making hard choices: Clarifying controversial ethical issues. *Journal of Counseling and Human Development, 19,* 1-10.

Sternberg, R. J. (2003). Responsibility: One of the other three Rs. *Monitor on Psychology, 34*(3), 5.

Stoltenberg, C. D., & Delworth, U. (1987). *Supervising Counselors and Therapists.* San Francisco: Jossey-Bass.

Stone, A. (1976). The Tarasoff decision: Suing psychotherapists to safeguard society. *Harvard Law Review, 90,* 358-378.

Stromberg, C. D., & Dellinger, A. (1993). Malpractice and other professional liability. *The Psychologist's Legal Update, 3.* Washington, DC: National Register of Health Service Providers in Psychology.

Stromberg, C. D., Haggarty, D. J., Leibenluft, R. F., McMillian, M. H., Mishkin, B., Rubin, B. L., & Trilling, H. R. (1988). *The Psychologist's Legal Handbook.* Washington, DC: The Council for the National Register of Health Service Providers in Psychology.

Stromberg, C., Schneider, J., & Joondeph, B. (1993). Dealing with potentially dangerous patients. *The Psychologist's Legal Update, 2.* Washington, DC: National Register of Health Service Providers in Psychology.

Studdert, D. M., Mellow, M. M., Gawande, A. A., Gandhi, T. K., Kachalia, A., Yoon, C., Puopolo, A. L., & Troyen, A. B. (2006). Claims, errors, and compensation payments in medical malpractice litigation. *The New England Journal of Medicine, 354,* 2024-2033.

Sullivan, T., Martin, W. L., Jr., & Handelsman, M. (1993). Practical benefits of an informed-consent procedure: An empirical investigation. *Professional Psychology: Research and Practice, 24,* 160-163.

Sutton, W. A. (1986, November 1). *Malpractice Issues in a Hospital Setting.* Workshop presented at CPC Parkwood Hospital, Atlanta, GA.

Switankowsky, I. S. (1998). *A New Paradigm for Informed Consent.* Lanham, MD: University Press of America.

Tarasoff v. Board of Regents of the University of California, 13 Cal.3d 177, 529 P.2d 533 (1974), vacated, 17 Cal.3d 425, 551 P.2d 334 (1976).

Thomas, J. L. (2002). Bartering. In A. A. Lazarus & O. Zur (Eds.), *Dual Relationships and Psychotherapy* (pp. 394-422). New York: Springer.

Tranel, D. (1994). The release of psychological data to nonexperts: Ethical and legal considerations. *Professional Psychology: Research and Practice, 29*(1), 33-38.

Tranel, D. (2000). Reply to the commentary on "Disclosure of tests and raw test data to the courts." *Neuropsychology Review, 10*(3), 177-178.

Twain, M. (1901, February 16). *Card Sent to the Young People's Society,* Greenpoint Presbyterian Church, Brooklyn.

Tymchuk, A. J. (1986). Guidelines for ethical decision making. *Canadian Psychology, 27,* 36-43.

Van Hoose, W. H., & Paradise, L. V. (1979). *Ethics in Counseling and Psychotherapy: Perspectives in Issues and Decision Making.* Cranston, RI: Carroll Press.

VandeCreek, L., & Knapp, S. (2001). *Tarasoff and Beyond: Legal and Clinical Considerations in the Treatment of Life-Endangering Patients* (3rd ed.). Sarasota, FL: Professional Resource Press.

Weiner, B. A., & Wettstein, R. M. (1993). *Legal Issues in Mental Health Care.* New York: Plenum.

Welfel, E. R. (2006). *Ethics in Counseling and Psychotherapy: Standards, Research, and Emerging Issues* (3rd ed.). Belmont, CA: Thomson Brooks/Cole.

White v. United States, 780 F. 2d 97 (D.C. Cir. 1986).

Whitree v. State, 56 Misc. 2d 693, 290 N.Y.S. 2d 486 (Ct Cl. 1968).

Wiger, D. E. (2005). *The Clinical Documentation Sourcebook: The Complete Paperwork Resource for Your Mental Health Practice.* Hoboken, NJ: John Wiley.

Williams, M. H. (2003). The curse of risk management. *Independent Practitioner, 23,* 202-205.

Woodsfellow, D. (2004). An ethics question: What do you think? *Georgia Psychologist, 58*(1), 19-20.

Woody, R. H. (1988). *Fifty Ways to Avoid Malpractice: A Guidebook for Mental Health Professionals.* Sarasota, FL: Professional Resource Exchange.

Woody, R. H. (1998). Bartering for psychological services. *Professional Psychology: Research and Practice, 30*(6), 607-610.

Younggren, J. N. (1995). Informed consent: Simply a reminder. *Register Report, 21,* 6-7.

Younggren, J. N. (2002a). *Ethical Decision-Making and Dual Relationships.* [Online]. Retrieved June 1, 2007, from http://www.kspope.com/dual/younggren.php

Younggren, J. (2002b, May 17). *Informed Consent, Record Keeping, and Accountability: Risk Management in the Era of HIPAA.* Continuing education workshop presented at the annual meeting of the Georgia Psychological Association, Savannah, GA.

Younggren, J. (2005, May 19). *APAIT Risk Management Workshop in Professional Psychological Practice.* APAIT ethics workshop presented at the annual meeting of the Georgia Psychological Association, Atlanta, GA.

Younggren, J. (2006, April 21). *Legal and Ethical Risks and Risk Management in Professional Psychological Practice: Risk Management in Specific High Risk Areas.* APAIT ethics workshop presented at the Georgia Psychological Association, Atlanta, GA.

Zuckerman, E. L. (2002). *The Paper Office, Third Edition: Forms, Guidelines, and Resources to Make Your Practice Work Ethically, Legally, and Profitably (The Clinician's Toolbox Series).* New York: Guilford.

Zuckerman, E. (2003). *HIPAA Help.* Pennsylvania: Three Wishes Press.

Zur, O. (2003). Is this HIPAA friendly: All you need to know about HIPAA's possums, ostriches, and eagles in three pages or less. *The Independent Practitioner, 23*(2), 79-82.

Subject Index

A

AACC. *See* American Association of Christian Counselors

AAMFT. *See* American Association for Marriage and Family Therapy

Abstinence, 65

Abuse
confidentiality exceptions for, 31, 32
emotional, 147
reporting adult, 144-145
sexual, 146

Abuse, child
definition of, 145-146
reporting, 87, 123, 144-148, 168

ACA. *See* American Counseling Association

ACA Ethical Standards Casebook (Herlihy/ Corey, G.), 84

Acting out, 165, 166

Actions
benefits and risks of, 91-92, 98-99, 156-157, 166
choosing course of, 100-101
consequences of, 87-88, 91-92, 98-99, 107, 117
developing alternative courses of, 97-98, 112
duties as, 87-88
easy *v.* ethical, 116
economics *v.* ethical, 117
entertainment *v.* ethical, 118
evaluating results of, 107
expediency *v.* ethical, 99, 117
extraversion *v.* ethical, 117-118
implementing course of, 106-107
pragmatism and practicality with, 99, 106, 117
principles and, 116-118
taking no, 97-98, 118-119
tests for, 98-99

Acts, commission and omission of, 121

ADD, diagnosing, 5

Addictive disease relapse prevention, 14

Adler, Alfred, 8

Administrative rule, 149

Advisory opinions, 114

Age of majority, 177-178, 179

Agency for Health Care Policy and Research (AHCPR), 18

AHAC. *See* American Home Assurance Company

AHCPR. *See* Agency for Health Care Policy and Research

American Association for Marriage and Family Therapy (AAMFT), 3, 141

American Association of Christian Counselors (AACC), 67, 71, 104-106

American Counseling Association (ACA)
Code of Ethics, 3, 51, 62-63, 64, 120-121, 164, 174
on consecutive therapy, 141
on disclosures, 149
on documentation/records, 129
on e-therapy, 159-160
on sexual impropriety, 62-63

American Counseling Association Ethical Standards Casebook (Herlihy/ Corey, G.), 4, 20, 109

American Home Assurance Company (AHAC), 65

American Professional Agency, 65

American Psychiatric Association, 3, 63, 120, 141

American Psychological Association (APA)
on child custody evaluations, 143-144
on competence, 7
on conflicts of interest, 57
on consecutive therapy, 141
on disclosures, 163
on documentation/records, 17, 124-129, 131-132, 136-138, 173-177, 182-183, 186, 187-188, 189-190

American Psychological Association *(Cont'd)*
on dual relationships, 47-49, 51-53
on duty to protect, 148-149
on ethical decision making, 83-85, 101-102, 109-110
on ethical violations, 164
Ethics Code, 3-4, 10, 22, 42, 51, 110, 114, 120-121, 149, 158-160, 169, 174, 190
on informed consent, 9-11, 27-31, 33-34, 36, 41-42
on sexual impropriety, 62
on terminating therapy, 157-158
American Psychological Association Insurance Trust (APAIT)
on communication, 18
on informed consent, 11, 32-33, 94
on projective retrospective thinking, 14
Psychotherapist-Patient Contract, 32-33, 38-39
American Psychological Association Practice Organization (APAPO), 135-136, 175, 181, 187
American Psychologist, 119
Anger Management, 6
APA. *See* American Psychological Association
APAIT. *See* American Psychological Association Insurance Trust
APAPO. *See* American Psychological Association Practice Organization
Aspirational obligations, 83, 199
Assent, as term, 27-28
Attorney, consulting with, 134, 135, 157, 168, 169, 173. *See also* Legal consultations
Autonomy, 84, 100-101

B

Bartering, for services, 72-75
Base rate effect, 155
Beneficence, 84, 100-101
Bentham, Jeremy, 87
Biofeedback, 6, 43
Biomedical ethical model, 100
Body language, 67
Boundaries
blurred, 58, 61
ego, 68, 71-72, 74, 76, 79-80
maintaining, vii, 2, 13-14
Boundaries, managing, 45-81, 194
points to remember, 81
summary of, 80-81

Boundaries, unhealthy
early warning signs of, 59-60
risk factors and, 59-61
Boundary crossings
nonsexual, 51, 60-61
violations *v.,* 45-46, 52, 60-61, 80, 139-140
Boundary Issues in Counseling: Multiple Roles and Responsibilities (Herlihy/Corey, G.), 53
Boundary violations
bartering and, 73
crossings *v.,* 45-46, 52, 60-61, 80, 139-140
Bradley v. Wessner, 149-150
Brainstorming, 97, 115, 119
Burnout, 165, 167
Business ethics, 86

C

California Board of Psychology, 73
Canadian Psychological Association (CPA), 93, 95, 96, 107
Canterbury v. Spence, 26, 36, 38
CAPS. *See* Christian Association for Psychological Studies
CAPTA. *See* National Child Abuse Prevention and Treatment Act
Case law, 149, 170, 184. *See also specific cases*
Categorical Imperative, in Formula of the Law of Nature, 87
Child custody evaluations
being aware of, 11-12
competence and, 6-7
consent forms for, 42, 43
consultations with colleagues on, 123, 143-144
performing, 5, 12, 113
tests in, 95
Child records, 177-180
conservative interpretation for, 178, 179
liberal interpretation for, 178-179
recommendations for, 180
Children
confidentiality and, 31-33, 37
informed consent and, 29, 36-38
parents and, 36-38, 95
parents and, in custody battles, 147-148
records for, 177-180
reporting abuse of, 87, 123, 144-148, 168

Christian Association for Psychological Studies (CAPS), 67-68, 71, 104-106
Client
  access, to records, 188-189
  blaming, 197
  concern for welfare of, 17, 41, 94, 99, 117, 118, 179, 180, 186, 198
  incompetent, consent for, 36
  patient *v.*, 3, 42
  physical contact with, 39, 69-72
  refusal of information by, 27
  satisfaction, therapist rating and, 26
  termination of noncompliant, 113, 123, 157-158
The Clinical Documentation Sourcebook: The Complete Paperwork Resource for Your Mental Health Practice (Wiger), 35
Clites v. Iowa, 38
Code of Conduct
  Georgia, 139, 151, 179, 180, 183
  Georgia Supplemental, 127, 160, 176, 177, 183, 184, 185-186
Code of Ethics for Psychologists (CPA), 93
Codes of Ethics
  AAMFT, 3
  ACA, 3, 51, 62-63, 64, 120-121, 164, 174
  commentaries on, 4
  for mental health professionals, 2-4
  NASW, 3, 64
Cognitive-behavioral therapy
  consequential thinking in, 14
  dialectical behavior therapy *v.*, 5
Collateral, informed consent of, 94
Commitment, involuntary, 29
Communication, viii
  informed consent and privileged, 134-135
  keeping open channels of, 18-20, 24
Community service agencies, role-blending and, 56
Competence(ies)
  consent for incompetent client, 36
  emotional, 7-8, 59
  informed consent and, 10, 28-29
  intellectual, 7
  involuntary commitment and, 29
  knowledge, 83, 106, 109, 169
  practicing within area of, vii, 2, 4-8, 11-12, 24, 194
  referrals and, 5-6
  skill, 83, 106, 109, 169
  technical, 5-7, 59
  training/guidelines for determining, 6-7

Complaints, ethics. *See also* Investigation
  behaviorism in responding to, 195-196
  characterological disturbance and likelihood for, 197
  documentation and unfounded, vii, 16, 24
  frivolous, 194-195
  notice of, 1-2
  points to remember, 202
  procedures and deadlines for, 199-200
  responding to, 193-202
  responding to, summary of, 201
  revealing name/nature of, 2, 16, 173
  understanding committee findings, 200
Confidentiality
  children and, 31-33, 37
  complete, 37, 135
  in couples counseling, 5
  duty to protect and, 15, 113
  exceptions to, 31-33, 103-104, 113, 156
  information release and, 123, 133-136
  informed consent and, 30, 31, 42, 111, 141-142
  limited, 37, 135
  with marriage and family therapists, 135
  no, 37, 135
  privacy, access to records and, 32
  privilege and, 4, 106
Conflicts checklist, 57, 74
Conflicts of interest
  bartering and, 74
  dual relationships and, 52, 56, 57, 59, 81
  questions regarding, 57
Consecutive therapy, 140-143
  Type I consecutive shift, 140-141
  Type II consecutive shift, 140-142
  Type III consecutive shift, 142-143
Consent. *See also* Informed consent
  forms, for child custody evaluations, 42, 43
  as term, 27-28
  voluntary, 28, 33
Consequences, of actions, 87-88, 91-92, 98-99, 107, 117
Consequential thinking
  in cognitive-behavioral therapy, 14
  ethical decision making and, 91, 99, 107, 115
Consultation, ethics. *See* Ethics consultations
Consultations
  legal *v.* psychological, 168-170
  peer, 15, 24, 36, 81, 100, 109, 113, 198-199

Consultations with colleagues, vii-viii, 2, 15-
        16, 23-24, 113-171
    on bartering, 74
    on child custody evaluations, 123, 143-
        144
    common dilemmas encountered during,
        116-118
    documentation of, 122, 170, 198-199
    on dual relationships, 48, 49, 56, 59, 81,
        90, 111, 123, 139-140
    ethical decision making and, 90, 91, 93,
        94, 95, 97-98, 101, 106, 111,
        194
    experienced *v.* less experienced, 115-116
    for high-risk situations, 15, 113
    informed consent and, 36
    points to remember, 171
    questions for, 4
    reasonableness and, 120-122, 170, 199
    on relationships, 48, 49, 56, 59, 81, 90,
        91
    summary of, 170-171
    top 10 reasons against, 118-120
    top 10 reasons for, 120-168
Continuing education, 6
Convergent thinking, 97
Counselors
    Code of Ethics for, 3-4
    smart *v.* wise, 15, 113
Couples counseling, 123, 140-143
    confidentiality in, 5
    informed consent in, 134-135
    records requests and, 134-135
    role-blending and, 140-141
    shifts between individual and, 140-143
Court orders, confidentiality exceptions by,
        32
CPA. *See* Canadian Psychological
        Association
Custody battles, parents and children in, 147-
        148
Cybercounseling, 158-160

D

Damages, 121
Deceased persons, records of, 130-131, 135-
        136
Decision making. *See* Ethical decision
        making
Defense mechanisms, psychological, 165-
        167
Denial, 165, 166
Deontological ethics, 86-88

Deposition, subpoena to take a, 133
Dialectical behavior therapy, 5, 7
Diminished capacity, 151
Direct or proximate cause, 121
Disclosure(s)
    client- *v.* therapist-oriented, 65-66
    discretionary, 31
    education, training and, 162-163
    of information, 187-188
    informed consent for, 163
    intimacy levels and, 65-68
    laws, 149
    mandatory, 31
    nonverbal, 67
    optional or negotiated, 31-32
    patient harm from, 35-36
    to protect, 148-149
    response *v.,* subpoenas and, 133-134
    as term, 27-28
    therapist, 65-69
Divergent thinking, 97
Divorce
    records requests and, 134
    reporting abuse and, 145, 148
Documentation, 173-191. *See also* Notes;
        Record(s); Record keeping; Record
        retention; *specific organizations*
    of consultations with colleagues, 122,
        170, 198-199
    of ethical decision making, 122
    explaining what you did and why you
        did it, 16, 17, 128, 184, 191,
        196
    importance of, vii, viii, 2, 194
    of informed consent, 10, 28, 34-35, 41-
        44
    points to remember, 191
    summary of, 191
    unfounded complaints and, vii, 16, 24
    written, 16-17, 24, 34-35, 189-191
*Documentation Standards for Behavior
        Treatment Records* (Magellan
        Behavioral Health), 183
Dolls, Anatomically Detailed, 6
Donaldson v. O'Connor, 184
Dual relationships, 46-59. *See also* Dual
        roles; Multiple role relationships
    conflicts of interest and, 52, 56, 57, 59,
        81
    consultations with colleagues on, 48, 49,
        56, 59, 81, 90, 111, 123, 139-
        140
    ethical decision making and, 54-55, 139
    exploitation and, 51, 53, 55, 56, 81, 90,
        140

Dual relationships *(Cont'd)*
  informed consent and, 55
  literature on, 53-55
  nonsexual, 54, 73, 139
  questions regarding, 54-55, 139
  role compatibility and, 90
  sexualized, 45
Dual Relationships and Psychotherapy
    (Lazarus/Zur), 51-52, 54
"Dual relationships: What's wrong with
    them?" (St. Germaine), 53
Dual roles
  concurrent and consecutive, 49-51, 58,
    140-143
  defined, 47
  foreseeable and unforeseeable, 48-51,
    58, 81, 123, 140
  normalization of, 51-53
Duty(ies)
  actions as, 87-88
  dereliction of, 121
Duty to protect
  confidentiality and, 15, 113
  third party, from harm, 115, 123, 148-
    157
Duty to warn, 148-153, 156-157

E

Economics, ethical actions *v.,* 117
Education, training and, 5, 6-7, 25, 65, 66,
    123, 142, 162-163
Egocentrism, 86
Electronic media, Internet and, 123, 158-160
EMDR. *See* Eye Movement Desensitization
    and Reprocessing
Emergencies, informed consent exception
    for, 35-36
Entertainment, ethical actions *v.,* 118
Errors, into amends, 198
E-therapy, 158-160
Ethical actions. *See* Actions
Ethical blind spots, 59, 81, 86, 96, 113, 171
Ethical Conflicts in Psychology (Bersoff),
    4, 20, 84
Ethical decision making, 83-112
  consequential thinking and, 91, 99, 107,
    115
  consultations with colleagues and, 90,
    91, 93, 94, 95, 97-98, 101, 106,
    111, 194
  documentation of, 122
  dual relationships and, 54-55, 139
  improving, 4

Ethical decision making *(Cont'd)*
  knowledge and proficiency in, 83
  multicultural diversity and, 94-95, 99
  points to remember, 112
  principles and, 83-85, 88, 95, 197
  proactive approach to, 110, 112
  questions about, 88-90, 94-101, 115
  reasonableness in, 107, 199
  steps in, 4, 115-116
  summary of, 111-112
  surveys on, 101-106
  values and, 89, 96, 116
Ethical decision-making models, viii, 24, 94-
    107
  assuming responsibility for consequence
    of actions in, 107
  basic, 88-94
  choosing course of action in, 100-101,
    112
  common features of, 93, 112
  considering community standards in,
    101-106
  considering personal biases, stresses,
    and self-interest in, 95-97
  considering possible risks and benefits
    in, 98-99
  developing alternative courses of action
    in, 97-98, 112
  evaluating results of action in, 107, 112
  four-step, 91-92
  identifying affected parties in, 94-95
  implementing course of action in, 106-
    107
  multistep, 92-94
  one-step, 88-89
  reactive approach of, 25, 110, 111, 112
  solution-generating/brainstorming
    approach to, 97, 115, 119
  three-step, 89-90
  two-step, 89
Ethical dichotomies, common, 115-118
Ethical no-brainer, 142
Ethical principles, 83-85
  actions and, 116-118
  guidelines to, vii-viii
  of informed consent, understanding, 27-
    28
*Ethical Principles of Psychologists and
    Code of Conduct* (APA/1992), 51,
    136
*Ethical Principles of Psychologists and
    Code of Conduct* (APA/2002), 3,
    10, 53, 84-85, 199. *See also* Ethics
    Code, APA
Ethical risk management. *See* Risk
    management

Ethical self-awareness, 59, 85, 96
Ethical standards, 84-85
    conflicts between legal and, 108-109,
        168, 171, 196
    understanding, 3-4
*Ethical Standards for Internet On-Line
    Counseling* (ACA), 159-160
Ethical violations/problems
    preventing, vii-viii, 23-24, 25, 43-44,
        110-111
    reporting, of colleagues, 124, 163-165
    responding to, in organizations, 124,
        165-167
Ethics Code, APA, 3-4, 10, 22, 42, 51, 110,
    114, 120-121, 149, 158-160, 169,
    174, 190
Ethics codes. *See* Codes of Ethics
Ethics committees
    adjudicatory role of, 114, 163-164
    advisory role of, 114, 163-164
    as colleagues *v.* adversaries, 195
    roles of, 113-115, 163-164, 195
    state professional associations, vii, 113,
        119, 123
    understanding findings of, 200
Ethics complaints. *See* Complaints, ethics
Ethics consultations, 68, 97-98. *See also*
    Consultations with colleagues
    legal *v.*, 168-170
    requesting, 15, 109, 113-115, 123
    supervision *v.*, 161-162
*Ethics for Psychologists: A Commentary on
    the APA Ethics Code* (Canter et al.),
    4, 20, 84, 92-93
*Ethics in Counseling and Psychotherapy:
    Perspectives in Issues and Decision
    Making* (Van Hoose/Paradise), 92
*Ethics in Psychology: Professional
    Standards and Cases* (Koocher/
    Keith-Spiegel), 53
*Ethics in Psychotherapy and Counseling: A
    Practical Guide for Psychologists*
    (Pope/Vasquez), 54
Events, special, 77-80
    formal and informal, 77-79
    public and private, 77-79
Ewing v. Goldstein, 154
Excellence, aspiring to, viii, 20, 121
Executive Coaching, 7
Expediency, ethical actions *v.*, 99, 117
Experience
    consultations with colleagues and, 115-
        116
    judgment and, 201
    turning negative into positive through,
        201

Exploitation
    bartering and, 73, 74
    dual relationships and, 51, 53, 55, 56,
        81, 90, 140
Extraversion, ethical actions *v.*, 117-118
Eye contact, 67
Eye Movement Desensitization and
    Reprocessing (EMDR), 6

F

Factorial matrix approach, 91-92, 99, 166
Federal regulations. *See also* Health
    Insurance Portability and Account-
    ability Act (HIPAA)
    regarding informed consent, 39-40
    on record retention, 175-176
Fidelity, 84, 100
Financial arrangements/fees, for treatment,
    30-31, 32-33, 34, 41, 111
"Finding of No Violation," 200
Fishing expedition, 2
Florida, 63-64, 146
Forensic evaluations, 143-144. *See also*
    Child custody evaluations
Forensic Examination, 7
Four Ds of malpractice (duty/dereliction of
    duty/damages/direct or proximate
    cause), 121
Francis de Sales, St., 120
Friendship, 8
Furnishings, 67

G

Garner v. Stone, 150
*General Guidelines for Providers of
    Psychological Services* (APA), 126,
    182, 188
Georgia
    Code of Conduct, 139, 151, 179, 180,
        183
    on disclosures, 149-151
    on documentation/records, 127, 175-
        176, 177-180, 183-186, 188-
        189
    on dual relationships, 52-53
    Jurisprudence Examination, 109, 169
    Supplemental Code of Conduct, 127,
        160, 176, 177, 183, 184, 185-
        186
Georgia Psychological Association (GPA),
    115

Georgia Psychologist magazine, 3
Getting Ready for HIPAA: A Primer for Psychologists (APAPO), 135-136
Gifts, accepting, 75-76
GPA. *See* Georgia Psychological Association
GPA Psychologists' Toolbox: Strategies for Building and Maintaining a Successful Private Practice (Sauls et al.), 134
Guardianship Evaluations, 7
Guidelines for Child Custody Evaluations in Divorce Proceedings (APA), 143-144

H

Hammer clause, 52-53
Health Insurance Portability and Accountability Act (HIPAA), 28, 102
    on confidentiality exceptions, 32
    on documentation/records, 124-125, 129-131, 135-136, 138, 174-176, 177, 179, 180-181, 187-189
    on informed consent, 28, 39-40
    possums, ostriches, and eagles with, 39-40
    Privacy Rule, 39-40, 129, 180-181
High-risk situations
    consultations with colleagues for, 15, 113
    supervision during, 9
HIPAA. *See* Health Insurance Portability and Accountability Act
Hugging, 70-71
Humor, 165, 166
Huxley, Aldous, 201
Hypnosis, 43
Hypotheses, deductive reasoning for testing, 6

I

Imago Therapy, 7
IMEs. *See* Independent Medical Examinations
Immunity statutes, 153-154
In the Matter of the Accusation Against Leon Jerome Oziel, Ph.D., 73
Incidental encounters, 57-58
Independent Consultative Examinations, 131, 190

Independent Medical Examinations (IMEs), 190
Informal inquiry, 5, 194
Information
    client's refusal of, 27
    disclosure of, 187-188
    release of, 31, 123, 133-136, 190-191
    release of, authorization for, 187-188
    release of, to third party, 31, 123, 131-133, 135, 190-191
    significant, informed consent and, 10, 28, 29-33
Informed consent, 25-44, 194. *See also specific organizations*
    autonomy-enhancing model of, 27
    children and, 29, 36-38
    of collateral, 94
    competence and, 10, 28-29
    confidentiality and, 30, 31, 42, 111, 141-142
    in couples counseling, 134-135
    for disclosures, 163
    dispensing with, 113
    documentation of, 10, 28, 34-35, 41-44
    dual relationships and, 55
    for e-therapy, 160
    ethical principles of, understanding, 27-28
    exception for emergencies, 35-36
    failure to obtain, 38
    federal regulations regarding, 39-40
    forced, 37-38
    forms, 10-11, 28, 34-35, 38-39, 41-44
    four elements of, 10, 28
    Golden Rule of, 30, 33
    initial intake interview and, 26, 31
    managed care and, 9, 26, 33, 40-41, 43
    obtaining adequate, 9-11, 24
    overview of, 26-27
    points to remember, 44
    privileged communication and, 134-135
    procedures, viii
    question-answer approach with, 27, 31
    significant information and, 10, 28, 29-33
    substitute, 10, 35, 36-38
    summary of, 43-44
    for third-party requests for services, 132-133
    undue influence and, 10, 28, 33-34
    waiver for, 35
Initial intake interview, 26, 31
Innovations in Clinical Practice (Doverspike), 3

Insurance. *See also* Health Insurance
    Portability and Accountability Act
    (HIPAA)
  disclosure to, 31
  history of mental disorder treatment's
      impact on, 26
  managed care and, 40-41
  risk-management questions for, 168-170
  on sexual impropriety, 61
Intellectualization, 165, 166
Internet
  Addiction Disorder, 160
  electronic media and, 123, 158-160
Investigation
  closure of, 200, 201
  dismissing, 200
  notice of, 1-2, 193-194
  notice of, responding to, 194
Issues and Ethics in the Helping Professions
    (Corey, G. et al), 53

J

Jablonski v. United States, 150
Jaffee v. Redmond, 154-155
Jewelry, 67
Journal of Counseling and Development
    (Gibson/Pope), 85
Journalists, 118
Judgment
  experience and, 201
  mistakes and, 107
Justice, 84, 100
  test of, 99

K

Kant, Immanuel, 87
Kassenbaum-Kennedy bill, 39
Keeping Children and Families Safe Act, 145
*Keeping Up the Good Work: A Practitioner's
    Guide to Mental Health Ethics*
    (Haas/Malouf), 53-54, 94, 122

L

Law(s). *See also* Federal regulations; State
    laws
  case, 149, 170, 184
  disclosure, 149
  statutory, 149, 170
the Law
  ethics and, 124, 168
  psychology and, 109-110

Law & Mental Health Professionals: Florida
    (Petrila/Otto), 108, 168, 169
*Law & Mental Health Professionals:
    Georgia* (Remar/Hubert), 108, 168,
    169
Legal consultations, 168-170
Liability. *See also* Insurance
  indirect or vicarious, 8-9
  limits, for threat of violence, 153-154
  supervision and, 8-9
Life tasks, on wheel to wellness, 8
Love, 8

M

Malpractice claims/suits. *See also*
    Professional malpractice
  communication and, 18-20
  excitement of, 119
  reducing, 122
  study of, 22-23
Malpractice, Four Ds of, 121
Managed care
  anticipating problems with, 111
  on documentation/records, 183
  informed consent and, 9, 26, 33, 40-41,
      43
  insurance and, 40-41
  precertification for, 33, 40-41
  referrals and, 6, 41
  short-term crisis intervention philosophy
      of, 41
Managed care organizations (MCO), 56
Mandatory obligations, 83-84
Marriage and family therapists
  Code of Ethics for, 3
  confidentiality with, 135
MCO. *See* Managed care organizations
Medical Economics magazine, 194
Memory(ies)
  recovered, 43
  testing, referrals for, 5
Mental health professionals (MHP), 2-4
MHP. *See* Mental health professionals
Mill, John Stuart, 87, 99
Mistakes
  correcting, 198
  judgment and, 107
Moore, George, 96
Moral justification, types of, 86-88
Moral principles
  overarching, 84, 88, 99, 100-101, 156,
      198
  universal, 99

Moral thinking, 89
  critical evaluative level of, 89
  intuitive level of, 89
Multiple Relationships and Conflict of Interest for Mental Health Professionals: A Conservative Psycholegal Approach (Ebert), 54
Multiple role relationships, 46, 80-81, 89-90

N

Narcissistic Personality Disorder, 120
NASW. *See* National Association of Social Workers
National Association of Social Workers (NASW), 3, 64, 141
National Board for Certified Counselors (NBCC), 103
National Child Abuse Prevention and Treatment Act (CAPTA), 145-146
NBCC. *See* National Board for Certified Counselors
Negligence, professional, 121-122
Neutrality, therapeutic, 141, 142
Nonmaleficence, 84, 100, 198
Notes
  importance of, 16-17, 196
  process, 181
  progress, 14, 17, 34, 41, 123, 126-128, 181-184
  psychotherapy, 180-181, 189
  risk-managed, 184-185
  termination, 186
Notice, as term, 27-28

O

Obligations
  aspirational, 83, 199
  mandatory, 83-84
O.C.G.A. *See* Official Code of Georgia Annotated
Official Code of Georgia Annotated (O.C.G.A.), 129-131, 147, 177, 188-189
Omnipotence, 86
Omniscience, 86
Organizations, responding to violations in, 124, 165-167
Outpatient Treatment Reports (OTR), 41, 43

P

The Paper Office (Zuckerman), 35
Parents, children and, 36-38, 95, 147-148
Passive-aggression, 165, 166
Patient
  Bill of Rights, 28
  client *v.,* 3, 42
  criterion, 26
  dissociative, 5
  harm, from disclosure, 35-36
  -Psychotherapist Contract, APAIT, 32-33, 38-39
  rights, 40
Peer consultations, 15, 24, 36, 81, 100, 109, 198-199. *See also* Consultations with colleagues
Peer reviewers, 195, 196
People v. Poddar, 151
Period of uncertainty, 179-180
Personalities, principles *v.,* 101, 106, 117-118, 197
PhD (Psychologically High Deity), 120
PHI. *See* Protected health information
Photos, 67
Poddar, Prosenjit, 151-154
Posttherapeutic relationships, 62-64
Posttraumatic stress disorder, 194
Power differential, in relationships, 49, 55, 90
Prescriptions, forging, 167
Principle ethics, 85-86, 96. *See also* Ethical principles
Principles
  actions and, 116-118
  ethical decision making and, 83-85, 88, 95, 197
  moral, 84, 88, 99, 100-101, 156, 198
  personalities *v.,* 101, 106, 117-118, 197
The Principles of Medical Ethics With Annotations Especially Applicable to Psychiatry (American Psychiatric Association), 3, 63
Privacy, 32. *See also* Health Insurance Portability and Accountability Act (HIPAA)
Privilege
  confidentiality and, 4, 106
  exceptions to, 150, 154-155
  subpoenas and assertion of, 133
  therapeutic, 35-36
Problem-solving, viii, 83, 112, 139. *See also* Ethical decision making
Process notes, 181

Professional incest, 62-63
Professional malpractice, 121-122
Professional negligence, 121-122
Progress notes, 14, 17, 34, 41, 123, 126-128, 181-184
Projective retrospective thinking, 14-15
Protected health information (PHI), 39-40, 135
Prudence, 106
Psychiatrists, Code of Ethics for, 3-4
Psychological report, 186
Psychologists
    Code of Ethics for, 3
    competence guidelines for, 7
The Psychologist's Legal Handbook (Stromberg et al.), 28, 35, 108, 168, 169
Psychologist's Professional Liability Insurance Policy (APAIT), 11
Psychologist's Professional Liability Policy (AHAC), 65
Psychology
    Health, 7
    the law and, 109-110
Psychotherapy
    e-therapy v., 158
    notes, 180-181, 189
Publicity, test of, 99

R

Rationalization, 96, 165, 167, 195
Reasonableness
    consultation with colleagues and, 120-122, 170, 199
    in ethical decision making, 107, 199
Record(s). *See also* Child records; Health Insurance Portability and Account-ability Act (HIPAA); Summary of records
    access to, 32, 123, 125, 128-131, 138, 180, 188-189
    assessment, 186
    of deceased persons, 130-131, 135-136
    federal laws on, 135-136, 174, 188-189
    ownership of, 130
    requests, couples counseling and, 134-135
    state laws on, 135-136, 174, 176, 188-189
    storage costs for, 180
    treatment, 186-187
    withholding, for nonpayment of services, 138

Record keeping, 173-191. *See also* Documentation
Record Keeping Guidelines (APA), 124-127, 174-175, 182-183, 186
Record period, 177-178, 180
Record retention, 123, 124-125, 127
    adult records, recommendations for, 177
    federal regulations on, 175-176
    professional standards for, 174-175
    state laws on, 176
    summary of records and, 185-187
Recovered memories, 43
Referrals
    competence and, 5-6
    managed care and, 6, 41
    for memory testing, 5
Relationships. *See also* Dual relationships; Dual roles; Posttherapeutic relationships
    clarity of termination and, 90
    duration of, 49, 90
    hybrid, 51, 58-59
    power differential in, 49, 55, 90
    specificity of termination and, 49, 90
Reports
    psychological, 186
    written, 189-191
Resigning, 165, 167
Risk-managed notes, 184-185
Risk management
    curse of, 21-22
    myth of, 21-23
    personal reflections on, 1-24
    points to remember, 24
    reasons for practicing, 121
    summary of, 23-24
    worst of, 21, 23
Role(s). *See* Dual relationships; Dual roles; Multiple role relationships
    blurring/confusion, 56
    compatibility, 90
    of ethics committees, 113-115, 163-164, 195
Role-blending, 51, 53
    couples counseling and, 140-141
    supervision and, 55-56
Role-clarification, 142
Rolfing, 70
Rules of Georgia Composite Board of Professional Counselors, Social Workers, and Marriage and Family Therapists, 127-128

S

Schrader v. Kohut, 161-162
Self-assertion, 165, 167
Self-determination, 101
Self-direction, 8
Self-disclosures, therapist, 65-69
Sex claims, 61
Sexual abuse, 146
Sexual impropriety/misconduct, 13, 52, 61-65
Sexualized dual relationships, 45
Shoebox case, 45
Significant information, informed consent and, 10, 28, 29-33
Slippery slope phenomena, 60-61, 140
Social workers, Code of Ethics for, 3
Special requests, 77-80, 118, 139-140
Specialization
    competence and, 6-7
    definition of, 5
Spirituality, 8
Stakeholders, 94
Standards. *See also* Ethical standards
    citing, 196
    conflicts between ethical and legal, 108-109, 168, 171, 196
    considering community, 101-106
    keeping current with, vii
    overarching moral principles and, 84, 88, 100
State laws
    legal advice regarding, 2
    on records, 135-136, 174, 176, 188-189
State licensing boards
    inquiries by, 1-2, 32
    state professional associations *v.,* 114
State professional associations
    ethics committees, vii, 113, 119, 123
    Legal Service Plans, 168
    state licensing boards *v.,* 114
Stealth dilemmas, 59
Sublimation, 165, 167
Subpoenas
    to appear, 133
    to appear and produce, 133
    responding to, 123, 133-134
    to take a deposition, 133
Summary
    closing, 186-187
    discharge, 186-187
Summary of records, 185-187
Supervision
    concerns about, 123, 160-162
    consultation *v.,* 161-162

Supervision *(Cont'd)*
    ethics consultations *v.,* 161-162
    during high-risk situations, 9
    liability and, 8-9
    role-blending and, 55-56
Suppression, 165, 167

T

Tarasoff, Tatiana (Tanya), 151-154
Tarasoff threshold, 153
Tarasoff v. Board of Regents of the University of California, 151-154
Tarasoff warnings, 153
Teleological ethics, 86-88
Tennessee, 147
Termination
    clarity of, relationships and, 90
    of noncompliant client, 113, 123, 157-158
    note, 186
    specificity of, relationships and, 49, 90
Test(s), 98-99
    in child custody evaluations, 95
    memory, 5
    protocols, release of, 137
Test data
    release of, 123, 136-138
    six grounds for refusal to release, 137-138
    test materials *v.,* 138
Test materials
    requests for, 123, 136-138
    test data *v.,* 138
Therapeutic privilege, 35-36
Therapists
    in abuse validator role, 145, 147
    disclosures, 65-69
    marriage and family, 3, 135
    rating, client satisfaction and, 26
Third party
    duty to protect, from harm, 123, 148-157
    information released to, 31, 123, 131-133, 135, 190-191
    requests for services, 123, 131-133
the Three Cs (caring/concerned/conscientious), 198
Touch, 69-72
    acceptable forms of, 69-71
    questions regarding, 71-72
    unacceptable forms of, 69-70

Training
    education and, 5, 6-7, 25, 65, 66, 123,
        142, 162-163
    guidelines and, for determining
        competence, 6-7
Transparency, 65
Treatment
    alternative forms of, 30
    benefits, risks and limitations of, 30-31,
        34
    financial arrangements/fees for, 30-31,
        32-33, 34, 41, 111
    nature and course of, 31
    records, 186-187
Triangulation, 37, 135, 145, 147
Trust, 101, 156-157
Twain, Mark, 20, 83, 196
2 x 2 Factorial Matrix, 91-92, 99, 166

U

Undue influence, informed consent and, 10,
        28, 33-34
Universalistic hedonism, 87
Universality
    expediency *v.,* 106
    test of, 99
Utilitarianism, 87

V

Values
    ethical decision making and, 89, 96, 116
    self-disclosure and, 67
Veracity, 84, 101
Violations. *See* Boundary violations; Ethical
        violations/problems; "Finding of No
        Violation"
Violence. *See also* Duty to protect
    liability limits for threat of, 153-154
    predicting, 155-156
    warning about threat of, 87, 91-92
Virtue ethics, 85-86, 95-96
Visualization techniques, 96-97
    private, 96-97
    public, 96
Voice inflection, subtle, 67

W

Weapons effect, 155
White v. United States, 184
Whitree v. State, 184
Withdrawal, 165, 167
Work and leisure, 8
Worker's compensation, confidentiality
        exceptions and, 32

Z

Zur, Ofer, 21

Author Index

A

Ackerman, M. C., 12
Ackerman, M. J., 12
Acuff, C., 40
Alexander, B., 98
American Association for Marriage and Family Therapy (AAMFT), 3
American Counseling Association (ACA), 3, 51, 62-63, 64, 120, 129, 149, 159-160, 164, 174
American Home Assurance Company (AHAC), 65
American Psychiatric Association, 3, 63, 120
American Psychological Association (APA), 3-4, 9-10, 12, 17, 22, 27-31, 33-34, 36, 41-42, 47-49, 51-53, 57, 62, 64, 83-85, 94, 99, 100, 101-102, 108, 109-110, 114, 120-121, 124-129, 131-132, 136-138, 141, 143-144, 148-149, 157-160, 163, 164, 168-169, 173-177, 182-183, 186, 187-188, 189-190, 197-198, 199
   Committee on Professional Practice and Standards, 7
   Division 12 Section II and Division 20 Interdivisional Task Force on Practice of Clinical Geropsychology, 7
   Division 44/Committee on Lesbian, Gay, and Bisexual Concerns Task Force, 7
   Office of Ethnic Minority Affairs, 7
   Presidential Task Force on the Assessment of Age-Consistent Memory Decline and Dementia, 7
   Task Force on Sex Bias and Sex Role Stereotyping in Psychotherapeutic Practice, 7
American Psychological Association Insurance Trust (APAIT), 11, 14, 32-33, 94
American Psychological Association Practice Organization (APAPO), 135-136, 175, 181, 187
Anders, P. B., 156-157
Anderson, B. S., 135
Andrews, L. B., 34
Asimov, I., 95

B

Baird, K. A., 78, 140
Barnett, J. E., 25, 107
Barth, J. T., 136
Baruth, N. E., 30, 31, 34, 38
Bascue, L. O., 9
Bates, R. T., 124, 125, 175
Beauchamp, T. L., 100
Bednar, R. L., 122, 199
Bednar, S. C., 199
Behnke, S., 107, 110, 124, 125, 169, 170-171, 175, 199
Bennett, B. E., 4, 5, 8, 11, 14, 20, 25, 29, 30, 31, 32, 33, 34, 36, 38, 40, 71, 84, 92-93, 128, 133, 184, 197
Bentham, J., 87
Berkowitz, L., 155
Bersoff, D. N., 4, 20, 84
Boes, S. R., 8
Borys, D. S., 13, 61, 62, 69, 101, 102-103
Borzuchowska, B., 94
Bost, P., 18
Bricklin, P. M., 11, 34, 40
Bridge, P. J., 9
Bridges, J. D., 106
Brodsky, 63
Bryant, B. K., 20, 71

Buchanan, W., 106
Buckley, P., 63

C

California Civil Code, 153-154
Callanan, M., 4, 27, 32, 33, 35, 37, 42, 53,
    56, 60, 62, 72, 93, 125, 134, 158,
    175, 198
Campbell, E., 160-161
Campbell, L., 118
Canadian Psychological Association (CPA),
    93, 95-96, 98, 107
Canter, M. B., 4, 5, 20, 29, 33, 34, 36, 40,
    84, 92-93
Cartwright, B., 94
Charles, E., 63
Childress, J. F., 100
Cobia, D. C., 8
Committee on Ethical Guidelines for
    Forensic Psychologists, 7
Corey, G., 4, 8, 20, 27, 32, 33, 35, 37, 42,
    48, 53, 56, 60, 62, 72, 84, 93, 98-
    99, 108-109, 125, 134, 158, 175,
    198
Corey, M., 4, 27, 32, 33, 35, 37, 42, 48, 53,
    56, 60, 62, 72, 93, 125, 134, 158,
    175, 198
Courtney, J. C., 136
Craig, M. E., 144-145, 146
Crawford, R. J., 195-196

D

Day, J. D., 84, 100
DeFilippis, N. A., 106
Dellinger, A., 9, 13, 25, 26, 28, 29-30, 35-
    36, 38, 61
Delworth, U., 8
Dilts, R., 70
Doverspike, J. D., 17, 179
Doverspike, W. F., 3, 5, 6, 11, 17, 18-19, 23,
    24, 40, 41, 51, 54, 59, 61, 91, 93,
    96, 106, 121, 123, 128, 134, 144,
    153, 157, 170, 175, 177, 180,
    184-185, 194, 195, 199, 201
Dsurney, J., 106
Dull, V. T., 18

E

Eberlein, L., 4
Ebert, B. W., 54

Ellis, E., 12, 134, 145, 147-148
Eyde, L. D., 99

F

Federspiel, C. F., 18
Feldstein, M., 63
Felthous, A. R., 154
Finkelstein, M. M., 19
Fitzpatrick, M., 60
Fleer, J. I., 21
Florida Statutes, 146
Frankel, R. M., 18
Freudenberger, H. J., 8

G

Gabbard, G. O., 13, 45, 60, 62, 64, 139-140
Galvin, M. D., 26, 27, 31, 33, 34, 42
Gandhi, T. K., 22-23
Garcia, J., 94
Gartrell, N., 63
Gauld-Jaeger, J., 18
Gawande, A. A., 22-23
Georgia Psychological Association (GPA),
    115
Gibson, W. T., 67, 70, 71, 73, 75, 78, 85,
    101, 103-104, 122
Gilmour-Barrett, K., 93, 94, 100
Glaser, K., 4, 93, 101
Golden, L., 58
Gorawara-Bhat, R., 18
Gottlieb, M. C., 49, 64, 90, 139
Graves, J., 25
Greenberg, S. A., 12, 56, 143-144
Greenson, R. R., 65
Greenwood, A., 20, 71
Gutheil, T. G., 16, 17, 45, 128, 139-140, 185,
    198

H

Haas, L. J., 3, 4, 10-11, 27, 29, 30, 33, 53-
    54, 83-84, 93-94, 95, 96, 97, 99,
    100, 106-107, 108, 119, 122, 199
Haggarty, D. J., 11, 16, 28, 29, 30, 33-35,
    39, 108, 128, 168, 169, 181, 196
Hall, J., 25
Hall, J. S., 65
Handelsman, M. M., 26, 27, 31, 33, 34, 42
Harden, J., 4, 93, 101

Harrar, W. R., 8
Harris, E., 8, 11, 12, 14, 16, 20, 25, 27, 30,
        31, 32, 34, 38, 56, 122, 128, 133,
        144, 170, 181, 184, 197
Health   Insurance   Portability   and
        Accountability Act (HIPAA), 28,
        32, 39-40, 102, 124-125, 129-
        131, 135-136, 138, 174-176, 177,
        179, 180-181, 187-189
Herlihy, B., 4, 20, 37, 53, 84, 93, 98-99, 108-
        109
Herman, J. L., 63
Hickson, G. B., 18
Hill, M., 4, 72, 93, 101
Holroyd, J., 60
Homan, M., 165
Hubert, R. N., 29, 108, 133-134, 136, 168,
        169
Huxley, A. L., 201
Hyman, S. M., 58

J

Jones, S. E., 4, 5, 20, 29, 33, 34, 36, 84, 92-
        93
Joondeph, B., 155
Jourard, S. M., 65

K

Kachalia, A., 22-23
Kachigian, C., 154
Kalichman, S. C., 144-145, 146
Kant, I., 87
Karasu, T. B., 63
Keeping Children and Families Safe Act of
        2003, 145
Keith-Spiegel, P., 4, 6, 9, 53, 67, 70, 72-73,
        78, 85, 93, 94, 97, 98, 101-102,
        103, 106, 122-123, 125, 175
Kilburn, R. B., 8
Kingsbury, S. J., 119
Kirkland, K., 13, 61
Kirkland, K. L., 13, 61
Kitchener, K. S., 4, 89, 93
Kleemeier, B., 134
Kleemeier, C., 134
Knapp, S. J., 8, 9, 11, 17, 34, 40, 114, 156,
        196
Koocher, G. P., 4, 9, 53, 93, 94, 97, 98, 125,
        175
Kovacs, A. L., 18

L

Ladany, N., 9
Lamb, J., 18
Lambert, M. J., 199
Lankton, S., 70
Lawrence, G., 37
Lazarus, A. A., 23, 45, 48-49, 51-52, 54, 60
Lees-Haley, P. R., 136
Lehrman-Waterman, D., 9
Leibenluft, R. F., 11, 16, 28, 29, 30, 33-35,
        39, 108, 128, 168, 169, 181, 196
LePage, A., 155
Levinson, W., 18
Linehan, M. M., 5
Livermore, J., 155
Localio, R., 63

M

Magellan Behavioral Health, 183
Maheu, M. M., 160
Malmquist, C., 155
Malouf, J. L., 3, 4, 10-11, 27, 29, 30, 33, 53-
        54, 83-84, 93-94, 95, 96, 97, 99,
        100, 106-107, 108, 119, 122, 199
Marlatt, G. A., 14
Martin, W. L., Jr., 26
McCullough, J. P., Jr., 5
McGarrah, N. A., 147
McIntyre, T., 118-120
McMillian, M. H., 11, 16, 28, 29, 30, 33-35,
        39, 108, 128, 168, 169, 181, 196
McMinn, M. R., 68, 71, 101, 104-106
McRay, B. W., 68, 71
Meara, N. M., 84, 100
Meck, D., 118
Meehl, P., 155
Meek, K. R., 68, 71, 101, 104-106
Mellow, M. M., 22-23
Mill, J. S., 87
Miller, C. S., 18
Mishkin, B., 11, 16, 28, 29, 30, 33-35, 39,
        108, 128, 168, 169, 181, 196
Moldawski, S., 40
Molinaro, M., 9
Monahan, J., 155, 156
Moore, G., 96
Morris, R. J., 12
Mullooly, J. P., 18
Myers, J. E., 8

N

Nagy, T. F., 4, 5, 20, 29, 33, 34, 36, 84, 92-93
Nash, R., 98
Nathan, P. E., 8
National Association of Social Workers (NASW), 3, 64, 141
National Child Abuse Prevention Act of 1974 (CAPTA), 145-146

O

Official Code of Georgia Annotated (O.C.G.A.), 129-131, 147, 177, 188-189
Olarte, S., 63
Othmer, E. O., 6
Othmer, S. C., 6
Otto, R. K., 108, 168, 169

P

Paddock, J., 25
Paradise, L. V., 20, 92
Petrila, J. D., 108, 168, 169
Phelps, R., 40
Phipps, A., 134
Piazza, N. J., 16-17, 30, 31, 34, 38, 128, 184
Pichert, J. W., 18
Poizner, S., 93, 94, 100
Pope, K. S., 6, 10, 13, 15-16, 27, 54, 60, 61, 62, 64, 65, 67, 69, 70, 71, 72-73, 75, 78, 85, 89-90, 101-104, 106, 122-123
Preis, J. J., 124, 125, 175
Puopolo, A. L., 22-23

Q

Quaintance, M. K., 99

R

Rabinowitz, E. E., 69, 70
Randall, D., 93, 94, 100
Reaves, R. P., 13, 61
Remar, R. B., 8, 11, 14, 25, 29, 30, 31, 32, 34, 38, 108, 128, 133-134, 136, 153, 168, 169, 197

Remley, T. P., 4, 37, 93
Robinson-Kurpius, S. E., 37
Rolf, I. P., 70
Roter, D. L., 18
Rubin, B. L., 11, 16, 28, 29, 30, 33-35, 39, 108, 128, 168, 169, 181, 196
Rules of Georgia Composite Board of Professional Counselors, Social Workers, and Marriage and Family Therapists, 127
Rules of the State Board of Examiners of Psychologists, 52-53, 149, 178

S

Sanders, R. K., 63
Sauls, M., 118, 134
Saxton, J. W., 19
Schaffer, S. J., 110, 170
Schlosser, B., 11, 32, 38, 42
Schmidt, L. D., 84, 100
Schneider, J., 155
Shapiro, D. L., 12, 25, 30, 31, 34, 136
Shuman, D. W., 12, 56, 143-144
Sinclair, C., 93, 94, 100
Smith, D., 60
Smith, R., 25
Smith. R. S., 181, 187
Soisson, E. L., 17, 196
Sonne, J. L., 60
St. Germaine, J., 53
Stadler, H. A., 98
Sternberg, R. J., 86, 96
Stoltenberg, C. D., 8
Stone, A., 151
Stone, A. V., 157
Stromberg, C. D., 9, 11, 13, 16, 25, 26, 28, 29, 30, 33-36, 38, 39, 61, 108, 128, 155, 168, 169, 181, 196
Studdert, D. M., 22-23
Sullivan, T., 26
Sutton, W. A., 19
Sweeney, T. J., 8
Switankowsky, I. S., 27

T

Tabachnick, B. G., 6, 67, 70, 72-73, 78, 85, 101-102, 103, 106, 122-123
Terrell, C. J., 156-157
Thomas, J. L., 72
Thoreson, R. W., 8

Tower, R. B., 11, 32, 38, 42
Tranel, D., 136
Trilling, H. R., 11, 16, 28, 29, 30, 33-35, 39, 108, 128, 168, 169, 181, 196
Troyen, A. B., 22-23
Twain, M., 20, 83, 196
Tymchuk, A. J., 93, 98

V

Van Hoose, W. H., 20, 92
VandeCreek, L., 8, 9, 11, 17, 34, 156, 196
VandenBos, G. R., 20, 71
Vasquez, M. J. T., 10, 13, 27, 54, 60, 61, 89-90

W

Waite, D. R., 199
Webb, C., 24, 111, 160-161
Weiner, B. A., 25, 30
Welfel, E. R., 10, 93
Wettstein, R. M., 25, 30

Wiger, D. E., 35
Wilbanks, M., 106
Williams, M. H., 21-22, 23
Winston, S. M., 94
Witmer, J. M., 8
Wolgast, B., 9
Woodsfellow, D., 140-141
Woody, R. H., 74, 108

Y

Yeager, R. D., 16-17, 34, 38, 128, 184
Yoon, C., 22-23
Younggren, J. N., 8, 11, 12, 14, 18, 20, 25, 27, 30, 31, 33, 34, 40, 41, 42, 54-55, 56, 93, 144, 158, 170, 181, 184, 197

Z

Zuckerman, E. L., 35, 40
Zur, O., 39-40, 45, 48-49, 51-52, 54, 60

If You Found This Book Useful . . .

You might want to know more about our other titles and continuing education programs.

If you would like to receive our latest catalog, please return this form:

Name: _____
(Please Print)

Address: _____

Address: _____

City/State/Zip: _____
This is ☐ home ☐ office

Telephone: (_____)_____

E-mail: _____

Fax: (_____) _____

I am a:

☐ Psychologist   ☐ Mental Health Counselor
☐ Psychiatrist   ☐ Marriage and Family Therapist
☐ Attorney   ☐ Not in Mental Health Field
☐ Clinical Social Worker   ☐ Other: _____

☐ I am particularly interested in your continuing education programs.

◆   ◆   ◆

Professional Resource Press
P.O. Box 3197
Sarasota, FL 34230-3197

Telephone: 800-443-3364
FAX: 941-343-9201
E-mail: cs.prpress@gmail.com
Website: www.prpress.com

Add A Colleague To Our Mailing List . . .

If you would like us to send our latest catalog to one of your colleagues, please return this form:

Name: _____
(**Please Print**)

Address: _____

Address: _____

City/State/Zip: _____
This is ☐ home ☐ office

Telephone: (_____)_____

E-mail: _____

Fax: (_____) _____

This person is a:

☐ Psychologist   ☐ Mental Health Counselor
☐ Psychiatrist   ☐ Marriage and Family Therapist
☐ Attorney   ☐ Not in Mental Health Field
☐ Clinical Social Worker   ☐ Other: _____

Name of person completing this form: _____

◆   ◆   ◆

Professional Resource Press
P.O. Box 3197
Sarasota, FL 34230-3197

Telephone: 800-443-3364
FAX: 941-343-9201
E-mail: cs.prpress@gmail.com
Website: www.prpress.com